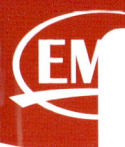

EMRA and ACMT

Medical Toxicology Guide

Editor-in-Chief
Kenneth D. Katz, MD, FACEP, FAAEM, FACMT
  Clinical Associate Professor
  University of South Florida Morsani College of Medicine
  Clinical Assistant Professor
  Philadelphia College of Osteopathic Medicine
  Department of Emergency and Hospital Medicine
  Lehigh Valley Health Network

Associate Editor
Ayrn D. O'Connor, MD, FACMT
  Member, ACMT Board of Directors
  Director of Medical Toxicology Fellowship
  University of Arizona College of Medicine Phoenix

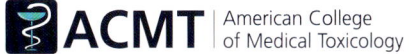

2018–2019 EMRA Board of Directors

President
Zach Jarou, MD

President-Elect
Omar Maniya, MD, MBA

Immediate Past President
Alicia Kurtz, MD

Secretary/Editor, *EM Resident*
Tommy Eales, DO

Speaker of the Council
Scott Pasichow, MD, MPH

Vice-Speaker of the Council
Nathan Vafaie, MD, MBA

Resident Representative to ACEP
Nida F. Degesys, MD

Director of Education
Sara Paradise, MD

Director of Health Policy
Rachel Solnick, MD

Director of Membership
Shehni Nadeem, MD

Director of Technology
Nick Salerno, MD

ACGME RC-EM Liaison
Eric McDonald, MD

Ex-Officio Board Member
Geoff Comp, DO, FAWM

Medical Student Council Chair
Sarah Ring

Staff
Executive Director
Cathey Wise, CAE

Managing Editor
Valerie Hunt

Disclaimer

This handbook is intended as a general guide to therapy only. While the editors have taken reasonable measures to ensure the accuracy of drug and dosing information presented herein, the user must consult other resources when necessary to confirm appropriate therapy, side effects, interactions, and contraindications. Use this guide in conjunction with advice from your regional poison control center and/or medical toxicologist. The publisher, authors, editors, and sponsoring organizations specifically disclaim any liability for omissions or errors found in this handbook, for appropriate use, or treatment errors. Further, although the publisher, authors, editors, and collaborating organizations have endeavored to make this handbook comprehensive, the vast differences in emergency practice settings may necessitate treatment approaches other than those presented here.

Copyright 2018, Emergency Medicine Residents' Association
ISBN 978-1-929854-51-6
4950 W. Royal Lane | Irving, TX 75063
972.550.0920 | emra.org

All rights reserved. This book is protected by copyright. No part of this book may be reproduced in any form or by any means without written permission from the copyright owner.

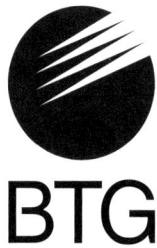

BTG is committed to promoting excellence in patient care and supporting medical education that is relevant to BTG's business and therapeutic areas. We support educational activities that are objective, balanced, and scientifically rigorous. To this end, we have provided an educational grant to support the publication of the *EMRA and ACMT Medical Toxicology Guide* in hope that it will benefit and facilitate the education of emergency medicine residents and their future patients.

Editors

Editor-in-Chief
Kenneth D. Katz, MD, FACEP, FAAEM, FACMT
Lehigh Valley Health Network

Associate Editor
Ayrn D. O'Connor, MD, FACMT
University of Arizona College of Medicine Phoenix

Medical Toxicology Editorial Team
Gillian A. Beauchamp, MD
Assistant Research Director, Section of Medical Toxicology
Lehigh Valley Health Network Department of Emergency & Hospital Medicine
Assistant Professor
University of South Florida Morsani College of Medicine

Robert D. Cannon, DO
Medical Toxicology Fellowship Program Director
Department of Emergency and Hospital Medicine
Lehigh Valley Health Network
Assistant Professor
University of South Florida Morsani College of Medicine

Matthew Cook, DO
Chief, Section of Medical Toxicology
Department of Emergency Medicine Section of Medical Toxicology
Lehigh Valley Health Network

Howard A. Greller, MD, FACEP, FACMT
Affiliated Medical Professor, Department of Clinical Medicine
CUNY School of Medicine
Director of Research and Medical Toxicology
Department of Emergency Medicine SBH Health Systems
St. Barnabas Hospital

A. Min Kang, MD, MPhil
Assistant Professor of Child Health and Medicine
University of Arizona College of Medicine—Phoenix

Louise W. Kao, MD, FACMT
Fellowship Director, Medical Toxicology
Associate Professor of Clinical Emergency Medicine
Indiana University School of Medicine

Kathryn Kopec, DO
Division Director, Medical Toxicology
Associate Professor of Emergency Medicine
Carolinas Medical Center, Atrium Health

Meghan B. Spyres, MD
Assistant Professor of Clinical Emergency Medicine
Department of Emergency Medicine
Division of Medical Toxicology
University of Southern California Keck School of Medicine

Evan S. Schwarz, MD, FACEP, FACMT
Associate Professor of Emergency Medicine
Medical Toxicology Section Chief
Washington University School of Medicine

Jerry W. Snow, MD
Assistant Professor of Emergency Medicine and Internal Medicine
Department of Medical Toxicology
Banner University Medical Center-Phoenix
University of Arizona College of Medicine

Ryan M. Surmaitis, DO
Department of Emergency Medicine and Medical Toxicology
Lehigh Valley Health Network

EMRA Reviewer
Sara Paradise, MD
Multimedia Design Education Technology Fellow
University of California, Irvine
Department of Emergency Medicine

Contributors

All contributors are affiliated with Lehigh Valley Health Network unless otherwise noted.

Faculty

Gavin C. Barr, Jr., MD
Eric W. Bean, DO, MBA
David B. Burmeister, DO, MBA
Michelle N. Carraro, DO
Richard Chow, DO
Gerald A. Coleman III, DO, FACEP
Amy L. Dunn, DO, MPH
Elizabeth M. Evans, DO
Jessica K. Eygnor, DO
Jeffrey M. Gesell, DO
Terrence E. Goyke, DO
Marna Rayl Greenberg, DO, MPH, FACEP
Jeanne L. Jacoby, MD
Steven A. Johnson, DO
Bryan G. Kane, MD, FACEP
Kathleen E. Kane, MD
Richard S. MacKenzie, MD, MBOE, FACEP
Andrew C. Miller, DO
Michael C. Nguyen, MD, FACEP
Shawn M. Quinn, DO, FACOEP, FACEP
Eileen C. Quintana, MD, MPH
David M. Richardson, MD, FACEP
Teresa M. Romano, MD, FAAP
Alexander M. Rosenau, DO, CPE, FACEP
Kevin R. Roth, DO, FACOEP
Mia J. Sclafani, DO
Joseph D. Sexton, MD
Kevin R. Weaver, DO, FACOEP
Charles C. Worrilow, MD
Susan K. Yaeger, MD

Emergency Medicine Residents

Osman Z. Abbasi, DO
Jamie Allen, DO
Alexandra M. Amaducci, DO
Ryan A. Anderson, DO
Kathryn B. Bartlett, DO
Smeet R. Bhimani, DO
Glenn A. Burket III, DO
Danielle L. Collins, MD
John W. Daubert, DO
Jessica Davis, DO
Ryan S. Day, MD
Zachary M. Dillon, MD
Kenneth Dzike, MD
Brittany J. Ely, DO
Joshua Enyart, DO
Erin Farber, DO
Rachel E. Fieman, MD
Derek J. Fikse, DO
Aaron S. Frey, DO
Julie A. Fritzges, DO
Victoria Goodheart, DO
Akshay Gupta, DO
Robert A. Gyory, MD
Kathryn A. Henry, DO
Michael R. Jong, MD
Priyanka Kailash, DO
Rafay A. Khan, DO
Emily A. Kiernan, DO
Andrew L. Koons, DO
Joseph Levi, DO
Jessica L. Maier, DO
Gregory A. Makar, DO
Matthew D. Marschall, DO
Wayne A. Martini, Jr., DO
Erica K. Mason, DO
Zachary M. Matuzsan, DO
Raymond J. Melder, Jr., DO
Andrew J. Miller, MD
Louis A. Morolla, DO
Matthew M. Palilonis, DO, MHSA
Pratik M. Parikh, DO
Claire L. Paulson, DO
Jennifer Sadowski, DO
Andrew W. Sheen, DO
Briana N. Tully, DO
Colleen E. Urban, DO
Hillary H. Ward, DO
Hanna R. Warren, DO
Kira D. Weaver, DO
Amy E. Wier, DO
Nathaniel M. Yoder, DO
Alexander Youngdahl, DO

Foreword

Welcome to the First Edition of the *EMRA and ACMT Medical Toxicology Guide*! The goal of developing this book is to provide the medical student, resident, fellow, and even seasoned attending practitioner a simple, clear, and pragmatic approach to the treatment of the poisoned patient at the bedside. Written by emergency medicine residents and attending physicians, the guide was then edited by a corps of experienced clinical and academic medical toxicologists to produce a stellar resource and the only guide of its kind. It is not meant to be an exhaustive tome to replace existing medical toxicology textbook reading but simply provide what you need to know—now. It is as evidence-based as possible and covers both uncommon and commonly encountered poisonings, envenomations, withdrawal states, and toxin exposures. Some recommendations must be made via consensus of the editors and their expansive knowledge base given that the field of medical toxicology sometimes lacks absolute evidence-based guidance; however, these recommendations are founded in the principle of attempting to be as judicious and thoughtful as possible to provide the best possible care of the poisoned patient—especially when action must be taken immediately to intervene and save lives. Moreover, the guide is also not meant to obviate direct communication with and recommendation from a medical toxicologist. The reader is strongly encouraged to contact the local medical toxicologist for guidance in conjunction with use of the book.

Our hope is that you find this book useful, and we welcome any feedback for future editions. Realize that we are all committed to taking care of the poisoned patient as optimally, efficiently, and in the best manner possible.

Acknowledgments

We would like to thank the following groups and people for their tireless efforts, without which this guide would not be possible: Lehigh Valley Health Network Emergency Medicine Residency Program; **Dawn Yenser**, **Manuel F. Colón**, BS, and **Marna Greenberg**, DO, MPH, CPE, FACEP, of Lehigh Valley Health Network; **Brian J. Levine**, MD, FACEP; **Jason Laskosky**, PharmD, BCPS; **Jamie Rosini**, PharmD, BCPS, BCCCP; and **Benjamin Abo**, DO, EMT-P, EMTT, FAWM. Special appreciation is extended to **Ayrn O'Connor**, MD, FACMT, and Charles McKay, MD, FACMT, and the American College of Medical Toxicology.

Dedication

This book is dedicated to my family, whose endless patience is unparalleled and forever appreciated.

Kenneth D. Katz
Editor-in-Chief

ACMT

My first encounter with medical toxicology was during medical school at Indiana University. I remember the passion and enthusiasm with which the medical toxicologists greeted every patient encounter and teaching opportunity. It was truly inspiring and I found myself drawn to this field because of this seemingly universal passion medical toxicologists have for teaching and for patient care. Now as a fellowship director and member of the American College of Medical Toxicology (ACMT) Board of Directors, my hope is that all students and residents will have an opportunity to work with a medical toxicologist rendering care at the bedside and improving patient outcomes.

It is with this hope in mind that ACMT eagerly accepted the opportunity to collaborate with EMRA and the many talented emergency physicians and medical toxicologists who contributed to this publication. Our unified goal was to provide a useful clinical tool to serve as a concise outline of common toxicologic exposures helping to guide care at the bedside with the additional hope of fostering the pursuit of deeper knowledge in the area of medical toxicology.

Medical Toxicologists and the care of the poisoned patient have come a long way. Gone are the days of giving strychnine or stimulants to patients suffering the toxic effects of CNS depressants or of inducing vomiting with syrup of ipecac. A focus on and improvements in supportive care have spurred drastic improvements in outcomes and mortality. Although the authors and editors of this guide must acknowledge that there are scenarios in which the evidence is limited or the science not fully elucidated leaving clinical care more nuanced, their collective clinical experience is so valuable in directing care. Additionally, one must recognize the constraints that such a succinct guide demands, meaning this publication should never replace discussing a clinical case with a medical toxicologist or your local poison center. Lastly, for those who find caring for these patients incites a deeper curiosity and interest, we hope you will consider further education in Medical Toxicology and know that ACMT will support you in your quest. Regardless of your career path we hope this guide serves you and your patients well.

Ayrn D. O'Connor, MD, FACMT
Member, ACMT Board of Directors

Glossary of Abbreviations

ABCDE: Airway, Breathing, Circulation, Disability/Dextrose, Exposure
ABG: Arterial blood gas
Ach: Acetylcholine
AchE: Acetylcholinesterase
AG: Anion gap
AKA: Alcoholic ketoacidosis
ARB: Angiotensin receptor blocker
ARDS: Acute respiratory distress syndrome
BAC: Blood alcohol content
BLL: Blood lead level
BMP: Basic metabolic panel (serum electrolytes, renal function)
CBC: Complete blood count
CDC: Centers for Disease Control & Prevention
CHF: Congestive heart failure
CMP: Comprehensive metabolic panel
CNS: Central nervous system
CO: Carbon monoxide
COPD: Chronic obstructive pulmonary disease
CPK: Creatinine phosphokinase
CSF: Cerebrospinal fluid
CV: Cardiovascular
CXR: Chest x-ray
DHP: Dihydropyridine
DIC: Disseminated intravascular coagulation
DMSA: Dimercaptosuccinic acid
ECHO: Echocardiogram
ECMO: Extracorporeal membrane oxygenation
EDTA: Ethylenediaminetetraacetate
EKG: Electrocardiogram
EMG: Electromyogram
FFP: Fresh frozen plasma
GABA: gamma-aminobutyric acid
G-CSF: Granulocyte colony-stimulating factor
GHB: Gamma-hydroxybutyrate
GI: Gastrointestinal
HAT: Heparin associated thrombocytopenia
HD: Hemodialysis
Hgb: Hemoglobin
HIT: Heparin-induced thrombocytopenia
HITT: HIT with thrombosis
HTN: Hypertension
ICP: Intracranial pressure
IDLH: Immediately dangerous to life and health
IVF: Intravenous fluids
LFT: Liver function tests
LMWH: Low molecular weight heparin
MALA: Metformin-associated metabolic acidosis
MAO/MAOIs: Monoamine oxidase/MAO Inhibitors
MDMA: 3,4-methylene-dioxymethamphetamine
MetHb: Methemoglobin
NADH: Nicotinamide adenine dinucleotide
NADPH: Nicotinamide adenine dinucleotide phosphate
NDRI: Norepinephrine dopamine reuptake inhibitor
NGT: Nasogastric tube
NH_3: Ammonia
NMDA: N-methyl-D-aspartate
NMJ: Neuromuscular junction
NMS: Neuroleptic malignant syndrome
NSS: Normal saline solution
N/V: Nausea, vomiting
N/V/D: Nausea, vomiting, diarrhea
PABA: Para-aminobenzoic acid
PCR: Polymerase chain reaction
PPE: Personal protective equipment
PPI: Proton pump inhibitors
PT/INR: Prothrombin time/international normalized ratio
PTT: Partial thromboplastin time
RBC: Red blood cell
SNRI: Selective norepinephrine reuptake inhibitor
SSRI: Selective serotonin reuptake inhibitor
TCA: Tricycle antidepressant
THC: Tetrahydrocannabinol
TSH: Thyroid-stimulating hormone
UA: Urinalysis
UFH: Unfractionated heparin
VBG: Venous blood gas
VPA: Valproic acid

Introduction

This on-shift guide is intended to help the clinician quickly identify and initiate treatment for the poisoned patient presenting to the emergency department. The goal is to provide clear direction as quickly as possible. Chapter organization is standardized so the user knows what type of information to expect, in what order.

This book is neither intended to replace existing toxicology textbooks, nor is it intended to address all nuances of toxicology. It serves as the initial reference for treatment but is not meant to be the only reference for complicated cases. When necessary seek guidance from local medical toxicologists or your regional poison control center.

Table of Contents

APPROACH TO THE POISONED PATIENT 1

ALCOHOLS
- Ethanol 9
- Ethylene Glycol. 11
- Isopropanol. 13
- Methanol. 14
- Propylene Glycol 17

BIOTERRORISM AGENTS
- Anthrax 19
- Botulism 21
- Plague. 23
- Radiation. .25
- Ricin 29
- Smallpox 31
- Tularemia .33

CAUSTICS
- Alkali. 35
- Hydrofluoric Acid 38
- Strong Acids (sulfuric, Hydrochloric) 36

ENVENOMATIONS/POISONINGS—MARINE

Envenomations
- Blue-Ringed Octopus. 43
- Cone Snail. 44
- Jellyfish ("true jellyfish") 45
- Box Jellyfish & Irukandji Jellyfish. 46
- Portuguese Man o' War 47
- "Scorpion Fish" Family (Lionfish, Scorpionfish, and Stonefish) 48
- Sea Anemone 50
- Sea Snakes 51
- Stingray. 52

Poisonings
- Ciguatera .53
- Scombroid. 55
- Tetrodotoxin 56

ENVENOMATIONS—NON-MARINE

Arachnids
- Black Widow. 57
- Brown Recluse 58
- Tarantula. .60

Hymenoptera
- Africanized Honeybees 60
- Fire Ants 62

Scorpions 63

Snakes
- Elapidae (Coral Snake) 65
- Viperldae (Pit Viper). 67

HEAVY METALS
- Arsenic/Arsine 73
- Iron 75
- Lead 77
- Mercury......................79
- Metal Fume Fever 81
- Thallium 82

HEMOGLOBINOPATHIES
- Carbon Monoxide..............85
- Methemoglobinemia 87

MUSHROOMS 91

PHARMACOLOGIC AGENTS
Acetaminophen 95
Anesthetics
- Local 99
- Nitrous Oxide 102

Antidysrhythmics
- Type I 103
- Type III....................107

Anticoagulants
- Direct Oral Anticoagulants (DOACs)....................108
- Heparin (Unfractionated, LMWH) and Antiplatelets 111
- Warfarin 113

Anticonvulsants
- Carbamazepine/Oxcarbazepine ..117
- Gabapentin 119
- Lacosamide 120
- Lamotrigine.................121
- Levetiracetam...............122
- Phenytoin 123
- Pregabalin 124
- Tiagabine 125
- Topiramate 126
- Valproic Acid...............127
- Vigabatrin 128
- Zonisamide..................129

Antidepressants
- Lithium 129
- MAOIs 131
- NDRIs, SNRIs, SSRIs........ 134
- Tricyclic Antidepressants (TCAs) 136
- Atypical Antidepressants: Bupropion..................139

Antidiabetics & Hypoglycemics
- α-Glucosidase Inhibitors 141
- Amylin Analog 142
- Biguanides 142
- DPP-4 Inhibitors 144
- GLP-1 Analogs...............144
- Insulin 145
- Meglitinides 147
- SGLT-2 Inhibitors 148
- Sulfonylureas 149
- Thiazolidinediones 150

Antihistamines & Antimuscarinics ...151

Anti-hypertensives
- ACE Inhibitors/ARB..........154
- α-1 Antagonists.............156
- α-2 Agonists 157
- β-Adrenergic Antagonists 159
- Calcium Channel Antagonists ...162
- Diuretics 165
- Vasodilators 165

Antipsychotics
- Typical..................... 167
- Atypical 170

Digoxin 172
Methotrexate 176
Methylxanthines (Caffeine, Theobromine, Theophylline) 178
Opioids 181
- Loperamide.................186
- Tramadol...................188

Salicylates................... 190

Sedative & Hypnotics
- Barbiturates 193
- Benzodiazepines 195
- Carisoprodol 196
- Baclofen 197
- Gamma-hydroxybutyrate (GHB). . 199
- "Z-Drugs" Imidazopyridine Hypnotic 200

PESTICIDES/RODENTICIDES
Pesticides
- Aluminum Phosphide 201
- Organophosphates & Carbamates 203

Rodenticides
- Barium 206
- Sodium Monofluoroacetate and Fluoroacetamide 207
- Strychnine 209
- Superwarfarins 210

PLANTS
- Ackee Fruit 215
- Antimuscarinic Plants 216
- Cardiac Glycoside Plants 217
- Cardiotoxic Na+ blockers 217
- Cardiotoxic Na+ Channel Openers 218
- Colchicine 219
- Hemlock—Poison 220
- Hemlock—Water 221
- Insoluble Oxalates 222
- Nicotine 222
- Pokeweed 223
- Toxalbumins 224
- Toxicodendron 225

SUBSTANCES OF ABUSE
Hallucinogens & Other Psychotropics
- Dextromethorphan 227
- Ketamine 228
- Lysergamides (Natural) 228
- Lysergic Acid Diethylamide (LSD) 229
- Mescaline 230
- Nutmeg 231
- Salvia 231
- Tryptamines (Indolealkylamines) 232

Marijuana
- Tetrahydrocannabinol (THC) ... 234
- Synthetic Cannabinoids 235

Nicotine 237
Sympathomimetics 238

SPECIAL SYNDROMES
Malignant Hyperthermia 243
Neuroleptic Malignant Syndrome 245
Serotonin Syndrome 247

TOXIC INHALANTS
Gases
- Chlorine 251
- Hydrogen Sulfide 252
- Nitrogen Dioxide 255
- Phosgene 256

WITHDRAWAL STATES
- Ethanol Withdrawal 259
- Opioid Withdrawal 264
- Sedative/Hypnotic Withdrawal (see Toxidrome Table, Appendix) 265

APPENDICES
- Common Formulas & Mnemonics 269
- Drug/Antidote Appendix 270

TOXIC THREATS 293

Approach to the Poisoned Patient

THINK LIKE A MEDICAL TOXICOLOGIST
- History
  - Medical
  - Psychiatric
  - Substance Use Disorder
    - Overdose
    - Withdrawal
  - Time last known well
  - Time of exposure and/or intent
  - Family/Friends
  - Social media
    - Texts
    - Pictures
    - Messages
- Environment
- Drug paraphernalia
- Prescriptions
  - Patient
    - Pharmacies
    - State drug database
    - Electronic records
- Maintain broad differential

   PEARL. Do not force diagnosis if doesn't fit

    - Infectious
    - Traumatic
    - Endocrine
    - Metabolic
    - Psychiatric

ABCDE

PEARL. Always priority, not gastric decontamination

- Airway
- Breathing
- Circulation
- Disability/dextrose
- Exposure

PHYSICAL EXAMINATION

- Vital Signs
  - Hyperthermia
    - Sympathomimetics
    - Salicylates
    - Serotonin syndrome
    - Dinitrophenol
    - Neuroleptic malignant syndrome
    - Sedative/hypnotic withdrawal
    - Malignant hyperthermia
    - Anticholinergics
  - Hypothermia
    - α-2 adrenergic agonists
    - Barbiturates
    - Carbon monoxide
    - Ethanol
    - Opioids
    - Sedative hypnotics
  - Tachycardia
    - Antidepressants
    - Antipsychotics
    - Sympathomimetics
    - Anticholinergics
    - Sedative/hypnotic withdrawal
    - Opiate/opioid withdrawal
    - Serotonin syndrome
    - Neuroleptic malignant syndrome
  - Bradycardia
    - Beta blockers
    - Calcium channel blockers
    - Cardiac glycosides
    - α-2 agonists
    - Organophosphates
    - Nicotine
  - Hypertension
    - α-1 adrenergic agonists
    - Antidepressants (not TCAs)
    - Antipsychotics
    - Sympathomimetics
    - Anticholinergics
    - Sedative/hypnotic withdrawal

- Opiate/opioid withdrawal
- Serotonin syndrome
— Hypotension
- Beta blockers
- Calcium channel blockers
- α-2 agonists
- α-1 antagonist
- Cyanide
— Tachypnea
- Salicylates
- Metabolic acidosis
— Bradypnea
- Opiates/opioids
- α-2 agonists
— Hypoxemia
- Opiates/opioids
- Noncardiogenic pulmonary edema
- Aspiration pneumonitis
- CNS
  — Pupils
  — Myoclonus
  — Tremor
  — Clonus
  — Hyperreflexia
- Derm
  — "Toxicology Handshake"
    - Anticholinergic vs. sympathomimetic toxidrome
    - Dry axilla: anticholinergic
    - Moist axilla: sympathomimetic
  — Track marks
  — Bullae
- Toxidromes (See Toxidrome Table, p. 282)
  — Cholinergics
  — Opioids/opiates
  — Sedative/hypnotics
  — Serotonin syndrome
  — Anticholinergic
  — Sympathomimetic
  — Neuroleptic malignant syndrome
  — Withdrawal states

DECONTAMINATION

PEARL. No role in majority poisonings and NOT a priority

PEARL. No proven mortality benefits

- Types and considerations
  - Activated charcoal
    - Preserved sensorium
    - Tolerate by mouth
    - Clinical deterioration not expected
    - No NGT
    - No sorbitol
    - Within 1-2 hrs
  - Gastric lavage
    - Witnessed, life-threatening poisoning
    - Within 1 hr
    - Intubate
    - Ewald tube (large-bore lumen tube)
    - Limited utility
  - Whole bowel irrigation
    - Life-threatening poisoning
    - Extended release
    - Enteric coated
    - Poorly absorbed by activated charcoal
      - Iron
      - Metals
      - Potassium
    - Drug packers
    - Polyethylene glycol
      - NGT
      - 2 L/hr
      - Clear rectal effluent
      - Limited utility

ANTIDOTES

PEARL. Know your hospital pharmacy supply

PEARL. Administer immediately those that can ameliorate or reverse imminently life-threatening poisonings (see Drug/Antidote Appendix, p. 270)

DIAGNOSTICS

PEARL. Routinely recommended for poisoned patient

- Serum chemistries
  - Rapid point of care testing if required immediately
  - Anion gap
- Acetaminophen
- Salicylate
- Ethanol
- Electrocardiogram
- Urinalysis
  - Ketones
  - Crystals
- Pregnancy test
- Common specifics
  - CPK
    - Rhabdomyolysis
    - Bullae
    - "Found down"
  - Lactate
    - Cyanide
    - Carbon monoxide
    - Metformin
    - Propylene glycol
    - Seizure
    - Ethanol related conditions
      - AKA
      - "Lactate gap"
        - Ethylene glycol
          - Serum (low or normal) vs. point of care (falsely elevated)
  - Serum osmolality
    - Toxic alcohols

    ### **PEARL.** Obtain serum ethanol and BMP at same time to calculate osmol gap

  - Carboxyhemoglobin
    - Winter
    - Enclosed spaces
    - Fire

- Methemoglobinemia
  - Persistent hypoxemia despite oxygen
  - Chocolate-colored blood
  - Cyanosis
  - Oxidizing agents
    - Benzocaine
    - Metoclopramide
    - Dapsone
- NH_3
  - Valproic acid
- Serum medication concentrations
- Common send outs
  - Volatile alcohol screen
  - Uncommon medications

PEARL. Know hospital laboratory capability

- Urine drug screen of abuse
  - Immunoassay
  - Limited clinical utility
  - Variable sensitivity/specificity depending on substance
    - THC and cocaine most specific
  - Requires confirmation

PEARL. Always treat the patient, never the drug screen

- Radiography
  - Trauma
  - Respiratory compromise
    - Aspiration pneumonitis
    - Non-cardiogenic pulmonary edema
      - Opiates
      - Salicylates

TREATMENT

PEARL. Meticulous supportive care paramount and mainstay of treatment in majority of poisonings

- Administer specific antidotes as indicated
- Reassess patient periodically
  - Clinical presentation changes
    - Medications absorbed, metabolized, or excreted
  - Response to antidotes or treatments
  - Repeat serum concentrations
    - Salicylate
    - Lithium
    - Valproate
    - Carbamazepine
  - Ask for help
    - Medical Toxicologist
    - Regional Poison Center

DISPOSITION

- Observe patients minimum 6 hrs
  - Monitored
- Extended or sustained release variable and unreliable onset of action and require longer period of observation or admission
  - Intentional, admit all
  - Unintentional or accidental depends on circumstances, drug, support and may be able to be discharged with thoughtful plan
- Admit
  - Critical illness
  - Progressively or persistently symptomatic
  - Rising serum medication concentrations
  - Patients requiring antidotal treatments

    PEARL. Admit those requiring > 1 naloxone dose

  - Intentional sustained or extended release ingestions
  - Poor home support
  - Elderly patients
  - Time of day
    - Children or elderly patients
    - Late evening or early morning

PEARL. "One Pill Can Kill"

- Pediatrics
  - Admit all:
    - Extended or sustained release calcium channel blockers
    - Extended or sustained release beta blockers
    - Extended or sustained release bupropion
    - Extended or sustained release venlafaxine
    - Oral hypoglycemic agents
    - Diphenoxylate/atropine
  - Strongly consider admission with following
    - Opioids/opiates
    - α-2 agonists
- Deeming medical stability for either home discharge or psychiatric evaluation
  - Asymptomatic or resolving signs/symptoms after observation
  - Declining serum concentrations and clinically stable
  - Improving or no diagnostic abnormalities

PEARL. NEVER MEDICALLY "CLEARED," ONLY MEDICALLY STABLE

Alcohols

ETHANOL

Sources
- Alcoholic beverages
- Less common exposure from mouthwash, perfume, cologne, aftershave, cooking extracts, OTC medications, hand sanitizers

Toxic Dose
- Variable and dependent on degree of tolerance in each individual

Mechanism of Action
- CNS depressant; synergistic with other depressants
- $GABA_A$ receptor agonist
- NMDA receptor antagonist

Clinical Manifestations
- Dose related
  - Affected by tolerance

  PEARL. Serum ethanol concentration does not reliably predict degree of clinical intoxication

- Mild intoxication
  - Disinhibition
  - Euphoria
- Moderate intoxication
  - Slurred speech
  - Impaired judgment/coordination
- Severe intoxication
  - Severely impaired coordination/judgment
  - N/V
  - "Black out" effects on memory
  - Hypothermia
- Life-threatening intoxication
  - Coma
  - Respiratory depression
  - Hypotension
  - Death

Diagnostics

- Good history and physical exam are paramount
  - Assessment for secondary/traumatic injury
- Serum ethanol concentration
  - Metabolism: Average clearance 20 mg/dL/hr; can be > 30 mg/dL/hr in chronic drinkers
- BMP
  - Hypoglycemia in pediatric or malnourished patients
  - Hypomagnesemia in chronic abuse
  - Hypokalemia
  - Hyponatremia in heavy beer drinkers with poor diets
  - AG acidosis in setting of AKA
    - If significant AG acidosis, check serum lactate and β-hydroxybutyrate
    - If severe or refractory AG acidosis, consider toxic alcohol intoxication
  - Contraction alkalosis in patients with repetitive vomiting
- LFT
  - AST:ALT = 2:1 in chronic alcoholics, and AST typically < 300 IU/L
- Serum lipase if pancreatitis is suspected
- Elevated lactate (can be marked in AKA)
- CBC
  - Macrocytosis
  - Thrombocytopenia

Treatment

- ABCDE
- Correct hypoglycemia
- Administer thiamine 200-500 mg, preferably IV
  - Higher doses for suspected Wernicke's encephalopathy
- Consider administration of folate/multivitamins
- Electrolyte replacement
- IV NSS for lactatemia associated with volume depletion
- Treat AKA with IV NSS, thiamine, IV dextrose, food

PEARL. Withdrawal may occur even if **BAC** is elevated (see Ethanol Withdrawal chapter, p. 259)

PEARL. Always consider concomitant medical or traumatic diagnoses, especially if clinical presentation does not fit ethanol intoxication

Disposition

- Admit
  - Moderate/severe or life-threatening intoxication
  - Persistent or worsening signs and symptoms

> **PEARL.** History of chronic abuse and multiple/severe prior withdrawal episodes may indicate greater risk for withdrawal. Prominent withdrawal symptoms may require hospital admission

- Concomitant morbidity (eg, acute pancreatitis, GI bleeding, traumatic injuries, etc.)

> **PEARL.** Recommend arranged transport home from ED

- Social work/counseling/rehabilitation referrals encouraged, especially for those with recidivism or combined psychiatric/drug abuse diagnoses

ETHYLENE GLYCOL

Sources
- Primary use as an automobile engine coolant (antifreeze)

Toxic Dose
- 95% 1-1.5 mL/kg

Mechanism of Action
- Ethylene glycol is metabolized to the toxins glycolate and oxalate via multiple enzymes, starting with alcohol dehydrogenase

Clinical Manifestations
- GI
  - N/V
- CNS
  - Inebriation
  - Cranial nerve palsies
  - Coma
- Renal
  - Acute kidney injury
  - Often late or delayed
  - Oxalic acid crystalluria

Diagnostics
- Serum ethylene glycol concentration (> 20 mg/dL toxic)
- BMP
- Serum ethanol concentration
- Serum osmolality (See Common Formulas, p. 269)

- UA

  PEARL. Urine fluorescence with Wood's lamp cannot clinically rule in or rule out ethylene glycol toxicity because of false negatives and false positives

- Lactate

  PEARL. Mind the "lactate gap"—difference between POC lactate (erroneously high because of glycolate cross-reactivity with L-oxidase reaction and serum lactate)

- ABG/VBG

Treatment
- ABCDE
- Fomepizole
  - Dosing
    - 15 mg/kg IV loading dose
    - 10 mg/kg IV q12hrs for 4 doses
    - 15 mg/kg IV q12hrs until cleared
      - ◆ Dose q4hrs during HD
  - Suspicion of ingestion plus any of the following:
    - pH < 7.3 (or low bicarbonate)
    - Osmol gap > 10 mOsm/kg
    - Anion gap > 12 mEq/L
    - Serum ethylene glycol concentration > 20 mg/dL
    - Serum ethanol concentration < 100 mg/dL
- Ethanol (if fomepizole unavailable)
  - Maintain blood ethanol concentration > 100 mg/dL
    - 8 mL/kg IV of 10% ethanol as a loading dose
    - 0.8-1.3 mL/kg/hr as maintenance or higher if ethanol tolerant or on hemodialysis

  PEARL. If sterile alcohol unavailable, give oral ethanol

- HD
  - Serum pH < 7.25 refractory to treatment
  - Signs of end organ damage: renal failure
- Adjunctive therapies
  - Sodium bicarbonate for severe or refractory metabolic acidosis
    - Bolus: 1-2 mEq/kg IVP over 1-2 min
    - Infusion: 100-150 mEq in 1 L D_5W @ 150-200 mL/h (2x maintenance in pediatrics)
  - Thiamine
    - 100 mg IV q6hrs
  - Pyroxidine
    - 50 mg IV q6hrs

Disposition
- Observe minimum 6 hrs, repeat labs
- Admit
  - High suspicion of ingestion
  - Severe, persistent, or worsening signs and symptoms or those requiring antidotal treatment
  - Ethylene glycol concentration > 20 mg/dL

ISOPROPANOL

Sources
- Rubbing alcohol
- Hand sanitizers
- Also used in topical pharmaceutical products, household, and cosmetic products

PEARL. Most common toxic alcohol exposure

Toxic Dose
- 0.5-1 mL/kg

Mechanism of Action
- Metabolized to acetone via alcohol dehydrogenase

Clinical Manifestations
PEARL. Ketosis without acidosis
- CNS
  - Inebriation
  - Coma
- CV
  - Tachycardia
  - Decreased peripheral vascular resistance
- GI
  - Fruity odor to breath from acetone
  - Abdominal pain
  - N/V
  - Hemorrhagic gastritis

Diagnostics
- Serum isopropanol concentration (if available)
  - Toxic concentration: 150 mg/dL

- Serum acetone concentration

> **PEARL.** Serum ketones can cause a false elevation in serum creatinine (can obtain point of care creatinine for comparison)

- BMP
- VBG/ABG
- Serum osmolality
- Serum ethanol concentration
- Serum or urine ketones
- EKG

Treatment
- ABCDE
- Supportive care
- May use PPIs for hemorrhagic gastritis
- Hemodialysis rarely indicated
  - If severe, life-threatening end-organ damage
  - Serum isopropanol concentration > 1000 mg/dL

Disposition
- Observe minimum 6 hrs
- Admit severe, persistent, or worsening signs and symptoms

METHANOL

Sources
- "Wood alcohol," mainly used as solvent in gasoline
- Moonshine
- Solvents
- Solid cooking fuel
- Racing fuel
- Paint removers
- Windshield wiper fluid

Toxic Dose
- 1 mL/kg

Mechanism of Action
- Methanol is metabolized to a toxic metabolite, formic acid, via alcohol and aldehyde dehydrogenase
  - Formate is mitochondrial poison leading to metabolic acidosis

Clinical Manifestations
- GI
  - N/V
  - Pancreatitis
- CNS
  - Similar ataxia, confusion, and slurred speech as ethanol, but less intoxicating than ethanol
  - CNS depression
  - Basal ganglia lesions
  - Putaminal necrosis with or without hemorrhage
- Ophthalmologic
  - Dilated pupils
    - Blindness/decreased visual acuity

    PEARL. "Snowfield vision" (disturbance resulting in small, flickering white dots in visual field)

    - Afferent papillary defect
    - Hyperemia of optic disc
    - Blurring of margins of optic disc
    - Central scotoma

Diagnostics
- Serum methanol concentration
  - Peak concentration 30-60 min after exposure
  - > 20 mg/dL toxic
- BMP
- ABG/VBG
- Serum osmolality (See Common Formulas, p. 269)
  - Osmol gap

    PEARL. A single calculation cannot be used to definitely exclude presence of toxic alcohol

    - Must calculate from sodium, glucose, blood urea nitrogen, and ethanol drawn at the same time as the serum osmolality
- Lactate
- Lipase
- Serum ethanol concentration
  - > 100 mg/dL may be protective due to blockade of alcohol dehydrogenase

Treatment

- ABCDE
- Fomepizole
  - Suspicion of ingestion plus any of the following:
    - Serum pH < 7.3 (or low bicarbonate)
    - Osmol gap > 10 mOsm/L
    - Anion gap > 12 mEq/L
    - Methanol concentration > 20mg/dL
    - Ethanol concentration < 100 mg/dL
  - Dose
    - 15 mg/kg IV loading dose
    - 10 mg/kg IV q12hrs x4
    - 15 mg/kg IV q12hrs until cleared
      - Dose q4hrs during hemodialysis
- Ethanol treatment (if fomepizole unavailable)
  - Maintain blood ethanol concentration > 100 mg/dL
    - 8 mL/kg IV of 10% ethanol as a loading dose
    - 0.8-1.3 mL/kg/hr as maintenance or higher if ethanol tolerant or on hemodialysis

    PEARL. If sterile alcohol unavailable, oral ethanol should be administered

- Metabolic acidosis
  - Sodium bicarbonate may be beneficial in keeping formic acid ionized and out of tissues, also consider for severe or refractory metabolic acidosis
  - IV sodium bicarbonate
    - Bolus: 1-2 mEq/kg IVP over 1-2 min
    - Infusion: 100-150 mEq in 1 L D5W @ 150-200 mL/h (2x maintenance in pediatrics)
- HD
  - Serum pH < 7.25 refractory to treatment
  - Signs of end organ damage
    - Vision disturbance
    - Renal failure
  - Consider for methanol concentration > 50 mg/dL, as clearance in presence of fomepizole is very prolonged
  - Avoid anticoagulation for HD because of risk of putaminal hemorrhage
- Adjunctive therapies
  - Folate: 1 mg/kg or 50 mg IV q4hrs
  - Thiamine: 100 mg IV QD

Disposition
- Observe minimum 6 hrs, repeat labs
- Admit
  - High suspicion of ingestion
  - Severe, persistent, or worsening signs and symptoms or those requiring antidotal treatment
  - Methanol concentration > 20 mg/dL

PROPYLENE GLYCOL

Sources
- Used as a solvent in many IV medications
  - Lorazepam
  - Phenytoin
  - Diazepam
  - Etomidate
  - Hydralazine

PEARL. Also used as a solvent in pharmaceuticals, "environmentally safe" antifreeze, and hydraulic fluid

Toxic Dose
- Lethal dose: > 10 g/kg
- IV medications > 25 mg/kg/day

PEARL. 0.1 mg/kg/hr IV lorazepam × 48 hrs associated with toxicity

Mechanism of Action
PEARL. Alcohol and aldehyde dehydrogenase metabolizes to lactate

Clinical Manifestations
- CNS
  - Coma
  - Seizures
- CV
  - Hypotension
  - Prolonged QRS
  - Bradycardia

  PEARL. Can be associated with rapid IV infusion
- Renal: acute kidney injury

Diagnostics
- Serum ethylene glycol concentration (if unknown "antifreeze" product)
- Serum propylene glycol concentration
  - Toxic concentration: 400 mg/dL reported in patient with severe toxicity
- Serum osmolality
- ABG/VBG
- Lactate
- BMP

Treatment
- ABCDE
- Discontinue medication administration if iatrogenic
- Fomepizole
  - Likely helpful
  - 15 mg/kg IV loading dose
  - 10 mg/kg IV q12hrs x4
- Metabolic acidosis
  - Sodium bicarbonate for severe or refractory acidosis
    - Bolus: 1-2 mEq/kg IVP over 1-2 min
    - Infusion: 100-150 mEq in 1 L D5W @ 150-200 mL/h (2x maintenance in pediatrics)
- HD
  - To reduce propylene glycol if worsening renal function

Disposition
- Observe minimum 6 hrs, repeat labs
- Admit
  - High suspicion of ingestion
  - Severe, persistent, or worsening signs and symptoms or those requiring antidotal treatment

Bioterrorism Agents

ANTHRAX

Source
- *Bacillus anthracis*: gram-positive, spore-forming bacteria
- High risk: farmers, ranchers, handlers of animal carcasses/hides/wools
- Types: Cutaneous, gastrointestinal, inhalational
- Most lethal route is inhalation of spores (most likely seen in bioterrorism)

Toxic Dose
- 2,500-50,000 spores

Mechanism of Action
- 3 components
  - Protective antigen
  - Edema factor
  - Lethal factor
- Inhalational
  - Aerosolized spores are phagocytosed by macrophages, then germinate
  - Transported to tracheobronchial lymph nodes where bacteria multiply
  - Not known to be transmitted person-to-person
- Cutaneous
  - Spores introduced in abrasions or skin openings
  - Majority of endemic cases
  - Bacteria multiply and form local infection or may disseminate
- Gastrointestinal/oropharyngeal
  - Rarer form
  - Ingestion of undercooked, contaminated meats
  - Direct ingestion; spores transported to local lymphatic tissue

Clinical Manifestations
- Inhalational: "Wool sorter's disease"
  - Incubation 1-7 days
  - Develop influenza-like illness
    - Fatigue
    - Malaise
    - Myalgia
    - Non-productive cough
    - Mild chest discomfort
    - Dyspnea

- Followed by rapid deterioration over next 24-48 hrs
  - Worsening respiratory distress
  - Bacteremia
- Sepsis
- Death within 24-36 hrs

PEARL. CXR demonstrates hemorrhagic mediastinitis, widened mediastinum

- Cutaneous
  - Papule develops 1-5 days after exposure
  - Lesions progress from macule to vesicle then ulcerate to form black eschar (necrotic) with surrounding edema
    - Eschar either sloughs off (illness resolved) or illness becomes disseminated with systemic symptoms (bacteremia, renal failure, anemia, bleeding) and death
- Gastrointestinal (2-5 day incubation)
  - N/V
  - Fevers
  - Malaise
  - Hematemesis
  - Hematochezia
  - Later symptoms: Hemorrhagic mesenteric lymphadenitis and ascites

Diagnostics

- CXR
- CBC
- BMP
- LFT
- Blood/sputum cultures
- Specialized testing available

Treatment

- ABCDE
- Infectious Disease consultation
- Antibiotics—60 days for mass casualty or post exposure prophylaxis
  - Doxycycline
  - Ciprofloxacin
  - Clindamycin
  - If severe PCN susceptible strain, amoxicillin or penicillin
- Inhalational
  - With meningitis: Dexamethasone, ciprofloxacin, meropenem, and linezolid

- Without meningitis: Ciprofloxacin or meropenem, plus clindamycin or doxycycline

For specific antibiotic dosing recommendations, please see the EMRA Antibiotic Guide

- Decontamination sporicidal/bactericidal solution
  - Spores can live for years in environment
- Droplet precautions unless aerosolized spores suspected (airborne/contact)
- Contact laboratory, local department of health, and CDC
- Hand washing over sanitizers (spores)
- Vaccine available for high risk professions and U.S. military

Disposition
- Admit all symptomatic patients

BOTULISM

Source
- Biotoxin produced by the bacteria *Clostridium botulinum*
- Spores can be found in food, soil, water
- No person-to-person transmission

Toxic Dose
- 0.01 mcg/kg inhalation; 70 mcg ingestion

Forms
- Foodborne (pre-formed toxin in undercooked food, honey, vegetables, canning)
- Wound
- Infantile
- Adult intestinal
- Iatrogenic
- Inhalational (most likely form in bioterrorism)

Mechanism of Action
- Heavy chain: Irreversibly binds presynaptic neurons
- Light chain: Cleaves various proteins, preventing the release of acetylcholine (Ach) from the presynaptic neuron
- Progressive descending motor paralysis with clear sensorium

Clinical Manifestations
- Foodborne
  - N/V
  - Cramping
  - Abdominal pain

- Constipation
- Progressive neurological symptoms
- Infantile "floppy baby"
  - Secondary to ingestion of spores, not to pre-formed toxin; immature gut allows for development of toxin
  - Often < 1 year old
  - 70% occur in breastfed infants
  - Constipation
  - Lethargy
  - Difficulty feeding
  - Altered cry
  - Neck weakness
- Wound
  - Contaminated wound
  - IV drug use/skin popping (black tar heroin)
  - Can have delayed presentation
  - The "D's"
    - **D**iplopia
    - **D**ysphonia
    - **D**ysphagia
    - **D**ysarthria
    - **D**ecreased deep tendon reflexes
    - **D**escending paralysis
  - Inhalational—progressive neurological symptoms
    - Dysarthria
    - Dysphagia
    - Ptosis
    - Diplopia
    - Mydriasis
    - Photophobia
    - Dysphonia
    - Progressive symmetrical descending paralysis
    - Diminished reflexes
- Onset of symptoms is dose-dependent

PEARL. Normal sensorium and afebrile

Diagnostics
- Send out tests available including:
  - ELISA
  - PCR
  - Mouse bioassays (blood, stool, or gastric samples/vomit)
- Electromyography shows reduced amplitude of motor potentials, but non-specific

Treatment/Infection Control
- ABCDE
- Negative inspiratory force: If < - 30 cmH$_2$0 consider intubation because respiratory muscles have been affected
- Wound debridement/antibiotics for wound botulism
- Contact laboratory, local department of health, and CDC
- Antitoxin available: trivalent, heptavalent, Baby BIG
  - Trivalent: Treats forms A, B, E
  - Heptavalent: Treats forms A, B, C, D, E, F, G
  - Goal to give as early as possible
  - Supplied by CDC
    - 10 cc vial diluted 1:10 in NSS and infused over 20 min IV
    - May repeat if needed
    - Inhibits circulating toxin, prevents progression
    - Does not reverse symptoms
    - Most efficacious in foodborne botulism (toxin possibly absorbed more slowly)
- Baby BIG
  - Human derived
  - Treats forms A & B

PEARL. Avoid aminoglycosides and clindamycin because of neuromuscular junction blocking effects

Disposition
- Admit all symptomatic patients

PLAGUE

Sources
- *Yersinia pestis*, gram-negative bacillus in 3 forms: bubonic, pneumonic, septicemic
- Transmitted through flea bites or inhalation; rodents (including prairie dogs), cats may be reservoirs for disease

Toxic Dose
- 100-500 organisms

Mechanism of Action
- Primary pneumonic plague: inhalational (bioterrorism)

  PEARL. Respiratory ISOLATION required
- Bubonic plague: inoculated into skin, such as by flea bite
- *Y. pestis* infects lymphatics and proliferates in lymph nodes causing necrosis; can subsequently cause sepsis by bacteremic spread

Clinical Manifestations
- Primary pneumonic (2-3 days after exposure)
  - Fever
  - Chills
  - Flu-like symptoms—cough, myalgias
  - Pneumonia
  - ARDS
  - Respiratory failure
  - Cardiovascular dysfunction
  - Up to 10% have plague meningitis
- Systemic toxicity includes:
  - Coagulation abnormalities and hepatocellular injury
  - DIC
- Bubonic plague (2-10 days inoculation period)
  - Buboes can be in groin, axilla, or cervical area
  - Fevers
  - Chills
  - Weakness
  - Headache
  - Malaise
  - Hepatomegaly
  - Splenomegaly
  - Gangrene of extremities/nose ("Black Death") secondary to coagulase enzyme in cooler areas of the body
  - 25% have vesicles or ulcerations at site of bite

PEARL. **Not recommended to I&D as lymphadenitis responds to antibiotics and can inoculate others**

- Historically 85% of cases are bubonic
- Can become disseminated: secondary septicemia plague (25%) or secondary pneumonic plague (transmissible to others; requires isolation)
- Primary Septicemia Plague: Inoculation from flea bite directly into blood stream
  - Gram-negative sepsis
    - Shock
    - High fevers
    - Rigors
    - Malaise
    - DIC
    - Petechiae
    - Endotoxemia
    - Death

PEARL. **KEY features of septicemia plague (primary or secondary)**
- Acral thrombosis
- Necrosis
- Gangrene of appendages ("Black Death")
— All forms of plague can disseminate into septicemia (secondary septicemia)

Diagnostics
- Gram stain and culture of sputum, blood, CSF, and aspirate from buboes (only if spontaneously draining) helpful
- CBC
- BMP
- DIC panel
- Blood cultures
- LFT
- CXR
- CDC or state health can use direct fluorescent antibody staining

Treatment
- **ABCDE**
- **Infectious disease consultation**
- Contact laboratory, local department of health, and CDC
- Antibiotics: 7-10 days
  — Ciprofloxacin
  — Doxycycline
  — Chloramphenicol
  — Streptomycin
  — Gentamicin
- Droplet isolation for pneumonic plague, for others use standard precautions
- Decontamination of surfaces is unnecessary, as plague cannot survive long outside of host

Disposition
- Admit all symptomatic patients

RADIATION

Sources
- Ionizing radiation
  — Electromagnetic waves (eg, Gamma (γ) and X-rays, and higher UV)
  — High-energy subatomic particles (eg, alpha (α) and beta (β) particles)
  — Sources:
    - XR

- CT
- Decay of radioisotopes
  - Nuclear meltdown
  - Dirty bomb
  - Food processing
  - Medical sterilization
  - Research laboratory
  - Environment (eg, radon)
- Irradiation means being exposed to ionizing radiation

PEARL. **Irradiated people/objects do not become radioactive**

- Contamination
  - External exposure to radioactive solids/liquids/droplets
  - Can lead to incorporation (into tissue, bone, thyroid, etc.)
- Alpha (α)
  - Travels short distances (1-2 cm) and does not penetrate skin
  - Can protect with paper or skin
  - Bad if inhaled
- Beta (β)
  - Penetrates up to a few layers of skin
  - Bad if inhaled or swallowed
- Gamma (γ) and X-rays
  - Pass through all layers of skin/tissue
  - Protect with shields

Isotope	α	β	Sources/Population at Exposure Risk
Americium-241	x		Ionization-type smoke detectors, oil exploration equipment, glass makers
Cesium-137		x	Medical equipment sterilization, radiation therapy, atomic clocks
Cobalt-60		x	Food/mail irradiation equipment
Iodine-131		x	Released during nuclear meltdown
Iridium-192		x	Cancer therapy
Plutonium-239	x		Thermoelectric generators, nuclear disaster
Radon-222	x		Found in basements, uranium miners
Tritium		x	Industrial workers, research labs
Uranium-233, 235, 238	x		Uranium miners, munitions factories

γ-rays are also produced in most α- or β- decays

Toxic Dose

- Dose estimator for exposure
  - Date/Time of exposure

- Date/Time onset of vomiting

PEARL. Calculator at https://www.remm.nlm.gov/ars_wbd.htm

- Vomiting within 1-5 hrs of exposure = likely exposure to > 6 Gy
  ≥ 6-16 Gy considered lethal even with supportive care
- Supralethal dose: ≥ 20 Gy
- 1 Gy (Gray): absorbed dose
- 1 Gy = 100 rad = 1 J/kg
  Ex: Abd CT= 2-5 rad; Head CT= 1 rad

Mechanism of Action
- Directly damages DNA
- Indirectly damages through free-radical formation (from XR, γ-rays) and cell structure damage

Clinical Manifestations
- Acute Radiation Syndrome
  - Constellation of signs and symptoms that develop after total body irradiation (thus requires penetrating radiation, or rarely, internal contamination)
    - GI (exposure > 6 Gy)
      - Early
      - N/V/D
      - Abdominal pain
    - Heme (exposure > 1 Gy)
      - Pancytopenia
      - Bleeding
    - CNS (exposure > 15-20 Gy)
      - Fatigue, headache
      - Hyperthermia
      - Hypotension
      - Neurocognitive deficits
      - Ataxia
      - Motor/sensory weakness
      - Seizures
      - Edema
    - Derm
      - Epilation (hair loss)
      - Erythema, edema, blistering, desquamation
      - Onycholysis
      - Abnormal sensation/itching

Diagnostics
- CBC

  PEARL. In those with persistent GI signs or symptoms, repeat CBC every 6 hrs; 48-hr lymphocyte count predicts mortality

- BMP
- Amylase
- C-Reactive Protein
- TSH (iodine)
- Specific tissue samples based on specific isotope encountered

Treatment
- ABCDE
- Follow standard trauma protocols
- Involve your hospital Radiation Safety Officer
- Radiation Emergency Assistance Center/Training Site (REAC/TS) at 865-576-1005
- Decontamination
  - Rescuers don standard personal protective equipment
  - Remove clothing with shears (Do NOT rip) = 90% of decontamination
  - Shampoo hair first, non-abrasive skin cleansing with soap/water
  - Irrigate wounds
  - Repeat until radioactivity is < 2x background activity
  - Consider gastric lavage and/or charcoal for ingestion of heavy metal
  - All materials including water need to be collected and disposed of appropriately
  - For Tx of ingestion/inhalation see Table on p. 29
- GI
  - IVF
  - Antiemetics/anti-diarrheal
- Heme
  - If late presentation
  - Blood products
  - G-CSF
- CV
  - IVF
  - Vasopressors

Isotope	Chelating/Blocking Agents (Adult) for Ingestion/Inhalation
Americium-241	Ca-DTPA, then Zn-DTPA: 1 g in 250 mL D5W IV over 30-60 min daily; Wounds: irrigate w/ 1 g DTPA in 250 mL H_2O
Cesium-137	Prussian Blue (low exposure burden): 500 mg PO q4hrs in 100-200 mL H_2O
Cobalt-60	May consider Ca-DTPA or Zn-DTPA: 1 g in 250 mL D5W IV over 30-60 min daily Wounds: irrigate w/ 1 g DTPA in 250 mL H_2O
Iodine-131	Potassium iodide: 300 mg PO immediately, then 130 mg PO (daily if not pregnant/breast-feeding)
Iridium-192	Gastric/bronchial lavage. Consider DTPA or EDTA
Plutonium-239	Ca-DTPA, then Zn-DTPA: 1 g in 250 mL D5W IV over 30-60 min QD; Wounds: irrigate w/ 1 g DTPA in 250 mL H_2O; (+/-) Aluminum-containing antacids for ingestion
Radon-222	Remove from source
Tritium	Copious IVF; consider HD
Uranium-233, 235, 238	$NaHCO_3$: 100 mEq in 500 mL of D5W by slow/constant infusion for alkalinization; (+/-) aluminum-containing antacids

Ca-DTPA or Zn-DTPA: calcium and zinc salt of diethylenetriamine pentaacetate

Disposition

- Admit symptomatic patients and those with clinical evidence of radiation poisoning, not simply external exposure/contamination

RICIN

Sources

- Protein derived from *Ricinus communis*, castor bean plant
- Byproduct of castor beans, which remains after castor oil extracted
- Occupational exposure in harvesting and processing plants
- Potential bioterrorism weapon
- Most potent if administered via parenteral or inhalational routes

Toxic Dose

- 5-20 mcg/kg injection

Mechanism of Action

- Induces cell death by inhibiting RNA synthesis
  — Binds to 60S ribosome
- Endothelial toxicity causes vascular leak
- Toxalbumin with 2 chains: A & B

Clinical Manifestations
- Based on route of exposure
- Inhalational
  - Direct toxicity to respiratory epithelium
  - Within 6 hrs
    - Fever
    - Cough
    - Congestion
    - Dyspnea
    - Arthralgia
    - Eye irritation
    - Nausea
  - No recorded fatal cases in humans but based on animal studies, expected signs & symptoms of end stage illness include:
    - Pulmonary edema
    - ARDS
    - Respiratory failure
    - Death
  - With smaller dose may get reactive airway disease or persistent asthma
- Ingestion
  - Symptoms
    - N/V/D
    - Abdominal pain
  - Higher doses
    - Necrosis of GI tract, liver, spleen, kidneys with systemic shock
    - Vascular collapse, shock

PEARL. Must chew ricin bean to cause toxicity (shell must be broken); whole ingested beans do not cause toxicity

- Parenteral
  - Intentional exposure (suicides, homicides, experimental)
  - Multi-organ system failure
  - Death

Diagnostics
- Confirmatory tests for ricin or ricinine require specialized laboratories
  - PCR
  - Gas or liquid chromatography
  - Radio assays
- CBC
- BMP
- LFT

Treatment
- ABCDE
- Decontamination for weaponized or inhaled ricin; ricin extremely stable
  - Proper respiratory protection
  - Denatures in heat > 80°F for 10 min
  - Remove clothing/jewelry
  - Wash with soap and water
  - Standard precautions after decontamination
- Contact laboratory, local department of health, and CDC
- Symptomatic treatment based on route of exposure
- If death occurs, usually within 3-4 days

Disposition
- Admit all symptomatic patients

SMALLPOX

Sources
- Variola virus, large DNA orthopoxvirus
  - Highly contagious—exposed skin, aerosolization
  - Eradicated in 1977
  - 30% fatality rate in unvaccinated population

Toxic Dose
- 100-500 organisms

Mechanism of Action
- Usually inhaled and enters oropharyngeal mucous membrane
- Multiplies in lymph nodes with subsequent viremia
- Patients with T-cell deficiencies are highly susceptible

Clinical Manifestations
- After 7-14 days incubation
  - Initial fever
  - Malaise
  - Myalgias
  - Weakness/fatigue
  - Backache
  - Headache
  - Ulcerative oropharyngeal lesions (shed virus into saliva)

- May have acute encephalopathy and abdominal pain
- 2-3 days following fever

> **PEARL.** Papular rash develops on face and spreads to extremities and trunk, likely to involve palms and soles

- Centrifugal distribution (trunk relatively spared)
- Rash progresses to vesicular, then deep pustular
- Rash scabs over 10-14 days after onset and leaves hypopigmented scars

> **PEARL.** Synchronous rash (all same stages of healing)

- Clinical variants may have:
  - Petechiae
  - Mucosal and dermal bleeding rather than classic rash
- If death occurs, usually during 2nd week of illness

Diagnostics
- Primarily clinical
- Specialized testing available
- Infectious Disease consultation
- Contact laboratory, local department of health, and CDC

Treatment/Infection Control
- ABCDE
- Cidofovir and ribavirin can be considered in outbreaks—must be given before symptoms start (within 2-3 days of exposure)
- Treatment is mainly supportive
- Consider vaccination—10 years of protection
  - Live vaccine from cowpox
  - Need to receive before infection or within first 2-3 days after exposure
- Respiratory isolation with negative pressure rooms, aerosol and contact precautions
- Infectious until all scabs fall off
- Contact hospital infection control, local and state health departments

Disposition
- Admit all symptomatic patients

TULAREMIA

Sources
- *Francisella tularensis*, aerobic, gram-negative *coccobacillus*
- Human transmission via arthropod bites (ticks, mosquitoes), consumption or handling of infected animal tissue or fluids (small mammals), or by inhalation of infective aerosols
- Not transmitted person-to-person

Toxic Dose
- 10-50 organisms

Mechanism of Action
- Exposure to animal body fluid
- Bite of tick or mosquito
- Aerosolization

Clinical Manifestations
- Abrupt onset
  — Fever (38-40°C)
  — Headache
  — Chills
  — Rigors
  — Myalgias (especially low back)
  — Coryza
  — Sore throat
  — N/V/D

  PEARL. Pulse-temperature dissociation with relative bradycardia

- Regardless of source of inoculation, may spread hematogenously, resulting in pleuropneumonia, septicemia, or meningitis
- Ulceroglandular tularemia: Inoculation into skin or mucous membrane
  — Focal infection and papule becomes centrally necrotic and tender, may have eschar
  — Spread to regional lymph nodes, intensely suppurative necrosis; lymph nodes may rupture
  — Local ulcer, lymphadenopathy, fever, chills, headache, malaise
  — May disseminate to other organs (10-15% develop pneumonia)
- Typhoidal tularemia: Inhalational inoculation, skin, or mucosal contact
  - Chest pain
  - Dyspnea
  - Rhabdomyolysis

- Pneumonia
- Renal failure
- Sepsis
- DIC
  - Distinct because no lymphadenopathy
- Pneumonic tularemia: Primary (inhalational) or secondary (hematogenous spread)
  - Hemorrhagic inflammation of the airways with
    - Hemoptysis
    - Bronchopneumonia
    - Respiratory failure
- Oropharyngeal: Inoculation usually through ingestion
  - Exudative pharyngitis
  - Cervical or retropharyngeal lymphadenopathy
  - Oral ulcerations
- Oculoglandular: Inoculation from ocular contact
  - Painful, purulent, or ulcerating conjunctivitis, usually unilateral
  - Periorbital edema
  - Preauricular lymphadenopathy
  - May lead to permanent conjunctival scarring

Diagnostics
- Specialized testing available of respiratory, blood, or tissue samples
- CBC
- BMP
- LFT
- Blood cultures
- CXR

Treatment
- ABCDE
- Consult infectious disease
- Contact laboratory, local department of health, and CDC
- Antibiotics
  - Doxycycline
  - Ciprofloxacin
  - Streptomycin
  - Gentamicin

Disposition
- Admit all symptomatic patients

Caustics

ALKALI

Sources
- Drain cleaners
- Lye
- Household and industrial strength bleach
- The concentration of the base is better predictor of corrosive effect than pH

Toxic Dose
- Higher concentration, volume, duration of exposure and pH > 12 increases risk of toxicity
- pH > 11-12 increases risk of injury

Mechanism of Action
- Dissociated hydroxide ions (OH-) penetrate tissues, causing necrosis

PEARL. Alkali agents cause liquefactive necrosis and penetration into deeper tissues

Clinical Manifestations
- Ophthalmologic/Derm
  - Usually causes immediate pain and redness, followed by blistering
  - Conjunctivitis and lacrimation common
  - Serious full-thickness burns and blindness may occur
- Ingestion
  - Dysphagia
  - Drooling
  - Stridor
  - Esophageal/gastric perforation
  - Mediastinitis
  - Hematemesis
  - Shock
  - Strictures are a late complication

Diagnostics
- CBC
- BMP
- CXR
- Endoscopy for ingestion
- Consider CT chest/abdomen/pelvis for suspected perforation after ingestion

Treatment
- ABCDE

PEARL. Do not attempt neutralization

- Immediate decontamination with copious irrigation for skin and eye exposures
- Inhalation
  - Secure airway early in patients with stridor, drooling, or other signs of respiratory compromise in anticipation of progressive airway obstruction or pulmonary edema/ARDS
  - Steroids are often used for airway edema
- Ingestion
  - Unintentional and minimal to no signs/symptoms
    - PO challenge with milk or water
  - Intentional, significant signs/symptoms or fails trial
    - GI consultation for endoscopy
    - Surgery consultation for suspected perforation

Disposition
- Admit
  - Intentional ingestions
  - Severe, persistent, or worsening signs and symptoms

STRONG ACIDS (SULFURIC, HYDROCHLORIC)

Sources
- Swimming pool cleaners
- Fertilizers
- Soldering fluxes
- Toilet bowl/ porcelain cleaner

Toxic Doses
- Higher concentration, volume, duration of exposure and pH < 2 increases risk of toxicity

Mechanism of Action
- HCl dissociates in water to form hydronium ions (H_3O^+) that can interact with tissue elements, resulting in cell injury or death
- Desiccation of epithelial cells results in eschar formation described as coagulation necrosis

Clinical Manifestations
- Inhalation
  - Irritation/inflammation (eyes, nose, respiratory tract)
  - Odor usually provides warning, but only 50% of exposed persons can perceive hydrogen chloride's odor
- Ophthalmologic/Derm
  - Severe burns, ulceration, scarring
  - Direct contact with aqueous solutions of HCl or with concentrated vapor can cause chemical burns
  - Hydrogen chloride is not absorbed through skin
- Ingestion
  - Corrosion of mucous membranes, esophagus, and stomach
  - Necrosis and perforation
  - Systemic toxicity may lead to metabolic acidosis

Diagnostics
- CBC
- BMP
- CXR for inhalation
- Consider CT chest/abdomen/pelvis for ingestion and suspected perforation
- Endoscopy for ingestion

Treatment
- ABCDE
- Decontamination
  - Remove clothing
  - Copiously irrigate exposed skin and eyes
- Inhalation
  - Administer supplemental oxygen
  - Treat bronchospasm if present with aerosolized bronchodilators
  - Consider racemic epinephrine for stridor
    - 0.25-0.75 mL of 2.25% racemic epinephrine solution in 2.5 cc saline, q20min PRN
  - Treatment with corticosteroids in high-dose exposures is controversial

- Derm
  - After irrigation, treat as thermal burn
- Ophthalmologic
  - Irrigate for at least 15 min or until pH of conjunctival fluid has returned to normal
  - Assess for corneal damage
  - Consult Ophthalmology if corneal damage present
- Ingestion
  - Unintentional and minimal to no signs/symptoms
    - PO challenge with milk or water
  - Intentional, significant signs/symptoms or fails trial
    - Surgery/GI consultation for endoscopy

Disposition
- Discharge accidental exposures who are asymptomatic and can tolerate PO
- Admit
  - Intentional ingestions
  - Severe, persistent, or worsening signs and symptoms

HYDROFLUORIC ACID

Sources
- Industrial
  - Concentrations may approach 100%
    - Etching/polishing glass
    - Pesticides
    - Plastics
    - High octane fuels
- Household
  - Concentrations typically 5-8%
    - Rust remover
    - Aluminum brighteners
    - Heavy-duty cleaners
- Route of exposure

PEARL. Any route of exposure can result in systemic toxicity

  - Derm
    - Most common exposure, usually the digits
    - Pain out of proportion to exam, frequently delayed presentation

- Inhalation
  - Severity ranges from mild airway irritation to severe burning and dyspnea
- Ingestion
  - Potentially fatal from systemic complications
- Ophthalmologic
  - Exposure to vapors or splash injury
  - Less likely to cause systemic complications
- Systemic
  - Complications arise from serious metabolic derangements because of fluoride anion

Toxic Dose
- Gas
  - 30 ppm IDLH
  - 5 min air exposure to 50-250 ppm can be fatal
- Solution
  - 50-70% very toxic and can cause immediate pain
  - Lower concentrations can cause less pain but more delayed tissue injury

Mechanism of Action
- HF is a weak acid that penetrates skin and soft tissue and binds Ca^{2+} and Mg^{2+} cations
  - Formation of CaFl and release of hydrogen ion results in tissue toxicity, pain, and electrolyte disturbances

Clinical Manifestations
- Derm
  - Onset of toxicity can vary by concentration
    - > 50% immediate pain and tissue destruction
    - 20-50% several hours before burns are apparent
    - < 20% may take 24 hrs before signs develop
  - Pain (often initially in the absence of physical findings)
    - Erythema
    - Discoloration
    - Systemic complications are anticipated with exposures involving large body surface area or high concentrations

PEARL. Symptoms may be delayed after exposure and skin findings do not correlate well with symptoms

- Inhalation
  - Hemorrhagic pneumonitis, ARDS, respiratory failure
  - Anticipate systemic complications
- Ophthalmologic
  - Corneal opacification
  - Corneal sloughing
  - Keratoconjunctivitis
  - Necrosis of anterior chamber
- GI (ingestion)
  - Caustic injury is not universal
  - N/V
  - Abdominal pain
  - Hemorrhagic gastritis
  - Shock
  - Systemic complications
  - High mortality rate
- Systemic
  - Severe refractory hypocalcemia
  - Hypomagnesemia
  - Hyperkalemia
  - Metabolic acidosis
  - Cardiac arrest because of refractory VFib and torsades de pointes
    - QT prolongation
    - Usually in setting of intentional ingestion or inhalation

Diagnostics
- Serial EKGs
- BMP
- CXR
  - Consider CT chest/abdomen/pelvis for ingestion or inhalation
- Endoscopy for ingestion

Treatment
- ABCDE
- Dermal injury
  - Decontamination
    - Remove clothing and irrigate with copious amounts of water
  - Topical calcium gluconate gel
    - Place 3.5 g calcium gluconate powder into 5 oz of water soluble gel and massage into skin or place in tight-fitting latex glove for at least 30 min

- Or 25 mL of 10% calcium gluconate and 75 mL of water soluble gel
- If pain unrelieved, consider digital block with lidocaine or bupivacaine
— Local subcutaneous infiltration of calcium gluconate
- Consider in burns with central gray area of coagulative necrosis, severe pain, or when topical therapy fails
- Using 27-30 gauge syringe, inject 0.5 mL of 10% calcium gluconate SQ for every square centimeter of burn
- Limited utility in digits due to volume restriction
■ Inhalation
— Early airway control anticipate evolution of ARDS
— Consider nebulized 4 mL of 2.5% calcium gluconate (1 mL of 10% calcium gluconate with 3 mL of normal saline)
- Limited evidence but no adverse effects reported
■ Ophthalmologic injury
— Copious irrigation with water, saline or LR (minimum 30 min)
— Cycloplegics for comfort

PEARL. Early Ophthalmology consult

■ Ingestion
— If ingestion < 1 hr, consider careful NGT placement and aspiration of gastric contents followed by gastric lavage using 10% calcium gluconate as diluent
— Consult surgery early due to risk of perforation
— Anticipate systemic toxicity
■ Systemic toxicity
— If significant exposure, IV calcium replacement should be started before lab results
- Adult: CaCl 10% (1 gm) IV over 10-15 min CENTRAL LINE ONLY; CaGluconate 10% (3 gm) IV over 5-10 min
- Pediatric: CaCl 10% 20 mg/kg IV over 10-15 min; CaGluconate 10% 20-50 mg/kg IV over 5-10 min, not to exceed adult dose
- Adult Infusion: 20-50 mg/kg/hr of $CaCl_2$ (10%), or 60-150 mg/kg/hr CaGluconate (10%)
- Administer CaCl via a central line due to risk of infiltration and subsequent tissue necrosis; calcium gluconate can be given peripherally
— IV MgSO4 2-4 g over 20 min
— Metabolic acidosis
- Isotonic sodium bicarbonate infusion

Disposition
- Admit
  - Intentional ingestion
  - Refractory pain
  - Severe, persistent, or worsening signs and symptoms or those requiring antidotal treatment

Envenomations/Poisonings—Marine

ENVENOMATIONS

Blue-Ringed Octopus

Sources
- Class *Cephalopoda*, phylum *Mollusca*
- *H. maculosa* (blue-ringed octopus)
- Found in tide pools and coral reefs commonly in the Indo-Pacific oceans

Venom
- Tetrodotoxin

Mechanism of Action
- Develop bright blue rings when threatened
- Small beak causes a puncture wound that releases tetrodotoxin
- Tetrodotoxin has Na^+ channel blocking effects

Clinical Manifestations
- Small puncture wounds with minimal pain initially
- Rapid progression
    - Paresthesias, perioral numbness
    - Paralysis
    - Fixed, dilated pupils
    - Respiratory arrest
- Patient is fully conscious while paralyzed
- Paralysis typically resolves within 24-48 hrs if patient survives

Diagnostics
- None

Treatment
- ABCDE
- Respiratory support
- Consider pressure immobilization bandage

Disposition
- Admit severe, persistent, or worsening sign and symptoms

Cone Snail

Sources
- Class *Gastropoda*, phylum *Mollusca*
- *C. geographus*
- Found in tropical & sub-tropical waters, mainly Indo-Pacific region

Venom
- Conotoxins

Mechanism of Action
- Hollow barbed radicular tooth stored in the proboscis delivers a potent venom containing conotoxins
- Conotoxins block Ca^{2+}, Na^+, K^+, and nicotinic ACh channels

Clinical Manifestations
- "Bee-like" puncture wound
- Local edema and cyanosis
- Mild cases
  — Localized paresthesias
  — Weakness
  — Nausea
- Severe reactions to envenomation
  — Paralysis
  — Bulbar palsy
  — Respiratory failure
  — Cardiac arrest

Diagnostics
- None

Treatment
- ABCDE
- Respiratory support
- Hot water (up to 45°C/113°F) immersion for 60-90 min for analgesia
- Adequate analgesia

Disposition
- Admit severe, persistent, or worsening signs and symptoms

Jellyfish ("true jellyfish")

Sources
- Class *Scyphozoa*, phylum *Cnidaria*
- Common syndrome: Sea bather's eruption
  - Thimble jellyfish (*L. unguiculata*)
- Found throughout most coastal waters

Venom
- Mixture of proteins, nonproteins, carbohydrates

Mechanism of Action
- Nematocyst apparatus for sting and venom discharge

Clinical Manifestations
- Mild stinging with local dermatitis and erythema
- Systemic toxicity extremely rare
- Resolution within hours

Diagnostics
- None

Treatment

PEARL. Sea water rinse and hot water

- Remove tentacles if present
- After tentacles removed, place hot water (up to 45°C/113°F heated to tolerance without burning) for pain relief for 60-90 min
- Consider
  - Topical lidocaine
  - Antihistamines
  - Corticosteroid cream
  - Analgesics

Disposition
- Admit severe, persistent, or worsening signs and symptoms

Box Jellyfish & Irukandji Jellyfish

Sources
- Class *Cubozoa*, phylum *Cnidaria*
- Contains some of the deadliest marine species
  - Hawaiian box jelly (*C. alata*)
  - Australian box jelly (*C. fleckeri*)
  - Irukandji jelly (*C. barnesii*)
- Mainly inhabit tropical waters, notably in the Indo-Pacific region

Venom
- Mixture of proteins, non-proteins, carbohydrates, cytolytic toxins

Mechanism of Action
- Nematocyst apparatus for sting and venom discharge
- Bell and tentacles of *C. fleckeri* may reach 30 cm and 3 m in length, respectively; bell and tentacles of *C. barnesi* are smaller, limiting detection in open waters
- Venom effects
  - Enhance Na^+ conductance
  - Enhance Ca^{2+} conductance
  - Catecholamines release
- Contains cardiotoxic properties, direct hemolytic, and necrotic properties

Clinical Manifestations
- Immediate severe pain
- Skin blistering/necrosis ("frosted ladder rash")
- Cardiac collapse
- Death can occur as quickly as 5 min after sting
- Irukandji Syndrome
  - Specific to Irukandji jellyfish
  - Caused by massive catecholamine release leading to:
    - Chest pain
    - Pulmonary edema
    - Severe hypertension
    - Cerebral edema
    - Cardiomyopathy
    - Heart failure

Diagnostics
- EKG

Treatment
- ABCDE
- 5% acetic acid rinse followed by tentacle removal
- Some evidence suggests hot water (up to 45°C/113°F) is effective in relieving pain (remains controversial whether hot water or acetic acid is most effective)
- Adequate analgesia
- Consider antihistamines and corticosteroids
- Consider antivenom for box jellyfish envenomation (where available) for:
  — Cardiac arrest
  — Respiratory distress
  — Cardiac dysrhythmias
  — Mental status changes
    - 1 vial IV, or 3 vials IM at 3 separate sites
- Irukandji Syndrome
  — In addition to the above, consider drawing cardiac enzymes and place on a cardiac monitor
  — BP control with phentolamine, magnesium, nicardipine, esmolol, or NTG
  — Consider short-acting titratable agents, as hypotension can occur

Disposition
- Admit
  — Severe, persistent, or worsening signs and symptoms or those requiring antidotal treatment

Portuguese Man o' War

Sources
- Class *Hydrozoa*, phylum *Cnidaria*
- Multi-organism colony
- Portuguese Man o' War (*P. physalis*) & Bluebottle (*P. utriculus*)
- Atlantic, Pacific, and Indian Oceans

Venom
- Mixture of proteins, non-proteins, carbohydrates, cytolytic toxins

Mechanism of Action
- Tentacles up to 30 m long, containing hundreds of thousands of venom-filled nematocysts

Clinical Manifestations
- Immediate localized pain
- Linear dermatitis
- Can progress to vesicles/bullae
- Necrosis
- Muscle spasm
- N/V
- Malaise
- Local numbness and paralysis
- Rarely hemolysis and acute kidney injury
- Symptoms typically resolve with 72 hrs

Diagnostics
- None

Treatment
- Seawater rinse

    PEARL. Standard treatment of *Physalia* species with acetic acid is controversial, as some studies have suggested it promotes nematocyst discharge

- Removal of tentacles
- After tentacles removed, place hot water (up to 45°C/113°F heated to tolerance without burning) for pain relief for 60-90 min
- Consider topical lidocaine, corticosteroid cream, and antihistamines as needed

Disposition
- Admit persistent or worsening signs and symptoms

"Scorpion Fish" Family (Lionfish, Scorpionfish, and Stonefish)

Sources
- Family *Scorpaenidae*
- Lionfish (*P. volitans*), scorpionfish (*S. plumieri*), and stonefish (*S. verrucosa*)
- Spiny fish found mainly in the tropical and temperate waters

Venom
- Serotonin, 5'-nucleotidase, phosphodiesterase, amino acids

Mechanism of Action
- Most to least toxic
  - Stonefish > Scorpionfish > Lionfish
- Venom contained in sharp, bony spines that run along the fish
- Various toxins have been isolated and shown to affect (primarily in animal models)
  - Ca^{2+} and K^+ channels
  - Acetylcholine release
  - Catecholamine release
  - Platelet aggregation
  - Vascular tone
  - Cardiac activity

Clinical Manifestations
- Local
  - Severely painful puncture wound
  - Local edema and cyanosis
  - Can develop blistering and necrosis

PEARL. Stonefish can cause severe systemic symptoms

  - Altered mentation
  - Fever
  - Nausea
  - Seizures
  - Paralysis
  - Pulmonary edema
  - Heart failure

Diagnostics
- Radiograph for foreign body

Treatment

PEARL. Hot water (up to 45°C) immersion for 60-90 min

- Adequate pain control
- Consider antibiotics for marine bacteria (*Vibrio* spp., *Pseudomonas* spp.)
- Surgical debridement if wound is extensive
- Stonefish antivenom in severe cases
  - 1-2 spine punctures: 1 vial IM
  - 3-4 spine punctures: 2 vials IM
  - \> 4 spine punctures: 3 vials IM
  - Epinephrine and diphenhydramine should be available if administering antivenom in case of allergic reaction

Disposition
- Admit severe, persistent, or worsening signs and symptoms or those requiring antidotal treatment

Sea Anemone

Sources
- Class *Anthozoa*, phylum *Cnidaria*
- Found along reefs and tidal pools

Venom
- Mixture of neurotoxic, hemolytic, cardiotoxic, cytolytic toxins

Mechanism of Action
- Nematocyst apparatus for sting and venom discharge
- Venom contains cytolytic and hemolytic toxins

Clinical Manifestations
- Local symptoms
  - Erythema
  - Pruritus
  - Blisters
  - Ulceration
- Systemic symptoms (rare)
  - Fever
  - Chills
  - Weakness
  - Nausea
  - Syncope

Diagnostics
- None

Treatment
- Seawater rinse, followed by topical 5% acetic acid
- Appropriate analgesia and wound care

Disposition
- Admit severe, persistent, or worsening signs and symptoms

Sea Snakes

Sources
- Family *Elapidae*
- Beaked sea snake (*E. schistosa*)
- Mainly in tropical waters of Indo-Pacific region
- Recent sightings off California coast

Venom
- Myotoxins, neurotoxins, hemotoxins, nephrotoxins
  - Acetylcholinesterase
  - 5'-nucleotidase
  - Phosphodiesterase
  - Phospholipase
  - Hyaluronidase
  - Leucine aminopeptidase

Mechanism of Action
- Venom causes:
  - Blockade at nicotinic acetylcholine receptors
  - Local hemolysis
  - Myotoxicity
- Approximately 20% of bites result in envenomation

Clinical Manifestations
- Relatively painless fang-sized bites
- If envenomation occurs
  - Rapid development of myalgia
  - Weakness
  - Blurry vision
  - Ascending paralysis
  - Rhabdomyolysis
- Severe symptoms can lead to
  - Acute renal failure
  - Respiratory arrest
- Respiratory paralysis may be delayed up to 6 hrs

Diagnostics
- CPK
- UA
- BMP

Treatment
- ABCDE
- Respiratory support
- Consider pressure immobilization bandage

> **PEARL.** Consider sea snake antivenom for any signs of envenomation because respiratory symptoms may be delayed

  — Usual dose: 1-3 ampules depending on severity and rapidity of envenoming; however, up to 10 have been used
  — If unavailable: tiger snake AV may be used; 1 vial sea snake AV = ~2-4 vials of tiger snake AV
  — Epinephrine and diphenhydramine should be available if administering antivenom

Disposition
- Admit all for 24 hrs for possible delayed neurotoxicity

Stingray

Sources
- Class *Chondrichthye*, Phylum *Chordata*
- Stingray (*D. dasyatis*)
- *Dasyatis Americana* common southeastern U.S.
- *Urolophus halleri* common western coast U.S.

Venom
- Mixture of serotonin, phosphodiesterase, 5'-nucleotides

Mechanism of Action
- Elongated, whip-like, barbed caudal appendage that harbors venom

Clinical Manifestations
- Localized puncture and laceration
- Local edema and cyanosis
- Moderate-severe pain
- Can cause local hemorrhage and necrosis
- Systemic symptoms (rare)
  — N/V
  — Cramps
  — Dysrhythmias
- Death from direct trauma
- Secondary wound infection may occur from retained foreign body

Diagnostics
- Radiograph for foreign body

Treatment
PEARL. Hot water immersion (up to 45°C) for 60-90 min
- Adequate pain control (IV or oral analgesics)
- Consider antibiotics
- Surgical management depending on extent & location of wound
    - Barb removal
    - Debridement
    - Wash out
    - Hemorrhage control

Disposition
- Admit severe, persistent, or worsening signs and symptoms

MARINE POISONING

Ciguatera

Sources
- May occur when eating large reef fish that containing ciguatoxin
    - Barracuda
    - Sea bass
    - Parrot fish
    - Red snapper
    - Grouper
    - Sturgeon

Toxic Dose
- 0.1 mcg ciguatoxin can cause poisoning in an adult

Mechanism of Action
- Ciguatoxin is a heat-stable, odorless, tasteless toxin produced by dinoflagellates (*Gambierdiscus toxicus*) and concentrated in carnivorous fish
- Ciguatoxin opens Na^+ channels

Clinical Manifestations
- Symptoms onset within 2-6 hrs
- CNS

  PEARL. Dysesthesia: Hot/cold temperature reversal

  — Paresthesias
  — Painful or loose-feeling teeth
  — Metallic taste
  — Tongue numbness
  — Paralysis
  — Seizures
- GI
  — N/V/D
  — Cramps
  — Dehydration
- CV
  — Bradycardia
  — Hypotension
- GI symptoms resolve in several days but CNS and CV symptoms may persist

Diagnostics
- None

Treatment
- Supportive care for GI symptoms and volume depletion
- Bradycardia: Atropine
  — **Adult**: 1-2 mg (mild) or 3-5 mg (severe) IV. Double q3-5min until dry. Maintenance load 10-20% of load IV qh, titrate PRN
  — **Pediatric**: 0.05-0.1 mg/kg (min 0.1 mg) IV. Double the dose if previous does not produce atropinization
- Consider amitriptyline, or gabapentin/pregabalin for prolonged neurologic symptoms (painful paresthesias)

Disposition
- Admit severe, persistent, or worsening signs and symptoms

Scombroid

Sources
- May occur when eating improperly stored fish
  - Tuna
  - Mackerel
  - Sardines
  - Mahi-mahi

Toxic Dose
- \> 100 mg of histamine per 100 g of fish

Mechanism of Action
- Bacterial growth on fish produces a heat-stable toxin: histidine decarboxylase

  PEARL. Toxin converts histidine to histamine and causes large histamine release when consumed

Clinical Manifestations
- Honeycomb appearance and peppery taste of fish sometimes reported
- Symptom onset within 1 hr
- Resolution in 8-12 hrs (without treatment)
- Flushing (predominantly on face and upper trunk)
- N/V/D
- Tachycardia
- Headache
- Pruritis
- Bronchospasm
- Can mimic allergic reactions

Diagnostics
- None

Treatment
- ABCDE
- Antihistamines
- Consider epinephrine and albuterol for severe respiratory symptoms

Disposition
- Admit severe, persistent, or worsening signs and symptoms

Tetrodotoxin

Sources
- Fish within the order Tetraodontiformes including pufferfish
- Frequently eaten in Japan, but gaining popularity in other locations
- Tetrodotoxin found in other animals, including blue-ringed octopus, horseshoe crab, newts, salamanders

Toxic Dose
- 1-2 mg of purified toxins can be lethal

Mechanism of Action
- Heat-stable toxin, tetrodotoxin, produces neurotoxicity by Na^+ channel inhibition
- Tetrodotoxin found primarily in liver, skin, ovaries, intestines

Clinical Manifestations
- Early symptoms (within minutes of ingestion)
  - Diaphoresis
  - Perioral paresthesias
  - Headache
  - N/V
  - Abdominal pain
- Later symptoms
  - Generalized weakness
  - Limb paresthesias
  - Cranial nerve dysfunction
  - Ascending paralysis (which can progress to respiratory arrest)
  - Hypotension
  - Cardiac dysrhythmias
- Delayed or improper treatment results in high mortality

Diagnostics
- None

Treatment
- ABCDE
- Supportive care
- Respiratory support

Disposition
- Admit all symptomatic patients

Envenomations—Non-Marine

ARACHNIDS

Black Widow Spider (Latrodectus mactans, Hourglass spider)

Source
- Red hourglass-shaped marking on ventral abdomen
- Found throughout North America except Maine

Mechanism of Action
- α-Latrotoxin
  - Causing presynaptic discharge of neurotransmitters (catecholamines and acetylcholines in particular)

Clinical Manifestations
- Local reaction
  - Minimal reaction, target lesion described as annular erythema with central clearing
  - Local diaphoresis
- Latrodectism
  - Widespread sustained muscle spasms/pain
  - Diffuse diaphoresis
  - Tachycardia
  - Flushing
  - Hypertension
  - N/V
  - "Pavor mortis" (fear of death)

  PEARL. Myopathic syndrome
  - Muscle cramps at the site of bite usually begin 15 min to 1 hr after the bite, progressing to muscle rigidity of large skeletal muscles (chest, abdomen, face)
  - Severe abdominal wall spasms may mimic an acute abdomen
  - Rare manifestations: priapism, acute cardiomyopathy, uterine contractions
  - *Facies latrodectismica*
    - Sweating
    - Contorted/grimaced face
    - Blepharitis, conjunctivitis, rhinitis
    - Periorbital edema

Diagnostics
- No confirmatory test
- BMP
- CPK
- EKG
- CXR if hypoxemic

Treatment
- ABCDE
- Pain/muscle spasm
  - Titrate benzodiazepines and opioids
  - Oral for mild cases and IV for more severe signs and symptoms
- Hypertension
  - If unresponsive once pain and muscle spasms are controlled with titration of opioids and benzodiazepines, can use direct vasodilators

  PEARL. Avoid β blockers; calcium and dantrolene not indicated

- Severe envenomation
  - *Latrodectus* antivenom (equine IgG antiserum) available for severe envenomations (acute cardiomyopathy, priapism, seizures, uncontrolled HTN, or threatened pregnancy loss)
  - Rapidly curative and effective but high risk of serum sickness and anaphylaxis
    - Contraindications include history of atopy (asthma, known allergy to horses)
    - 1 to 2 vials diluted in 100 mL D_5W or NSS infused over 1 hr

Disposition
- Admit severe, persistent, or worsening signs and symptoms or those requiring antivenom treatment

Brown Recluse (Loxosceles reclusa; Violin or Fiddleback Spider)

Source
- Violin shaped mark on dorsum of cephalothorax, 6 eyes
- South, Central, Midwest United States
- Envenomation unlikely outside endemic distribution

Mechanism of Action
- Cytotoxic
  - Sphingomyelinase-D and hyaluronidase

Clinical Manifestations

> **PEARL.** Necrotic arachnidism: serious dermal injuries characterized by local symptoms with increasing ulceration

- Days 1-3 central hemorrhagic ulceration surrounded by blanching ischemia and outer erythema (red/white/blue lesion)
- Days 3-4 progressive necrosis
- Days 5-7 eschar formation
- Days 7-14 eschar falls off and wound heals by secondary intention
- Loxoscelism
  - Rare systemic reactions
  - Hemolysis, coagulopathy, renal failure, DIC

Diagnostics

- No testing available to confirm acute diagnosis
- Loxoscelism
  - CBC
  - BMP
  - DIC panel

Treatment

- Supportive
  - Analgesia
  - Local wound care
  - Elevation
  - Update tetanus status
  - Severe wounds may require **delayed** surgical intervention

> **PEARL.** Avoid early excision because of possible ongoing tissue injury

- Antibiotics only indicated for secondary wound infection

Disposition

- Discharge
  - Local signs without systemic toxicity with outpatient serial wound re-examinations
- Admit
  - Loxoscelism, persistent, or worsening signs and symptoms or concern for secondary wound infection

Tarantulas

Source
- Large, hairy spiders
- Found in Southwest United States

Mechanism of Action
- Mixture of hyaluronidase, nucleotides, and polyamines causing local tissue injury
- Urticarial hairs contain chitin, lipoproteins, and mucopolysaccharides and cause irritation

Clinical Manifestations
- Bites are rarely harmful to humans; severe envenomation rare
- Urticarial hairs cause local histamine reaction with intense local inflammation and irritation
  - Involving skin, eyes, respiratory tract
  - Pruritus can persist for weeks

Diagnostics
- Slit lamp exam for ophthalmologic involvement

Treatment
- Remove hairs with tape
- Supportive care (analgesics, antihistamines, topical or systemic corticosteroids)
- Local wound care
- Tetanus prophylaxis for bites
- Ophthalmologic exam and removal of hairs

Disposition
- Discharge after supportive measures

HYMENOPTERA

Africanized Honeybees (Apis mellifera scutellata)

Source
- Africanized honeybee
  - Hybrid of African and European honeybee
  - They are more likely to swarm and their aggressiveness results in massive envenomation
  - Spread throughout Southern United States

Mechanism of Action
- Venom is a mixture of protein/polypeptide toxins, enzymes, and pharmacologically active low molecular weight compounds (histamine, serotonin, acetylcholine, dopamine)
- Melittin key component that disrupts cell membranes
- Phospholipase A_2 is immunogenic component and acts synergistically with melittin to destroy cell membranes

PEARL. **No significant difference between venom of Africanized honeybees and other bees but extreme quantity delivered due to multiple stings by African honeybee causes non-immune, non IgE, direct venom toxicity**

Clinical Manifestations
- Envenoming Syndrome
  - N/V/D
  - Hypotension
  - Tachycardia
  - Delayed
    - Rhabdomyolysis
    - Hemolysis
    - DIC panel
    - Acute kidney injury
    - Elevated LFT
    - Pancreatitis
    - Myocardial infarction due to demand ischemia
    - Shock
  - > 50 stings in an adult and > 1 sting/kg in children are associated with risk of systemic toxicity. Deaths in adults are reported in envenomations of > 500 stings
- Anaphylaxis can occur with just 1 sting and is distinct from massive envenomation

Diagnostics
- CBC
- CPK
- Troponin
- EKG
- BMP
- DIC panel

Treatment
- ABCDE

PEARL. Rapid removal of stingers is not necessary and there is no difference between pinching and scraping

  - Delayed stinger removal can be performed to reduce foreign body reaction
  - Remove dead bees from nares, ears, oropharynx
- Supportive care
  - Epinephrine infusion for shock, hypotension
  - Corticosteroids although not studied are thought to be useful in controlling edema that progresses over 24-48 hrs
  - Antihistamines (hydroxyzine or diphenhydramine)
- Anticipation and treatment of complications
  - Early intubation for airway edema
  - Hydration and monitoring of UOP (goal 2 cc/kg/hr) for rhabdomyolysis
  - Hemodialysis for acute renal failure

Disposition
- Consider 24 hrs observation for envenomation in children or adults at risk of delayed systemic toxicity

Fire Ants (Solenopsis invicta)

Source
- Fire ant
- Southeastern United States

Mechanism of Action
- 95-99% alkaloid (unique to the animal kingdom)
  - Cytotoxic, hemolytic, potentially cardiotoxic
- 1-5% immunogenic
  - Can sensitize an individual to the venom

Clinical Manifestations
- Pain
- Local wheal and erythema
- Development of sterile pustules within 24 hrs
- Can cause systemic symptoms, heart failure, and/or anaphylaxis if multiple stings or in a sensitized individual

Diagnostics
- None

Treatment
- Supportive care
  - Topical glucocorticoid ointments
  - Local anesthetic cream
  - Oral antihistamines
  - Local wound care
- Treat anaphylaxis

Disposition
- Admit severe, persistent, or worsening signs and symptoms

SCORPIONS

Sources
- *Centruroides sculpturatus* is the only scorpion in U.S. that produces clinically significant toxicity
  - Endemic to U.S. Southwest (Arizona, California, Nevada, New Mexico, Texas) and Mexico
  - Envenomations outside of normal geographical distribution rare
  - Yellow/straw to tan color with a tail that terminates in the telson
    - Containing a venom gland and stinger
  - Fatalities rare, but severe envenomations still occur
    - Most often in young children

Mechanism of Action
- Venom is a mixture of hyaluronidase, mucopolysaccharides, phospholipase, acetylcholinesterase, serotonin, histamine, protease inhibitors, protein neurotoxins, and histamine releasers
- Alters voltage-gated Na^+ channel inactivation
  - Producing increased sodium influx, prolonged duration and amplitude of action potentials and repetitive uncontrolled axonal firing of parasympathetic, sympathetic, and somatic neurons
  - Resulting in excessive catecholamine and acetylcholine release

Clinical Manifestations
- Envenomation
  - Sting characterized by sudden sharp, localized pain with burning and paresthesia
  - Symptom onset immediate, with progression over several hours

> **PEARL.** Local inflammatory signs absent or minimal with Centruroides sting

- Grading System
  - I Local pain and paresthesia at sting site
    - (+) Tap test—gentle tapping at sting site elicits pain/paresthesias
  - II Local AND remote pain and paresthesia
  - III Either neuromuscular hyperactivity or cranial nerve dysfunction
  - IV Both neuromuscular hyperactivity or cranial nerve dysfunction
    - Neuromuscular hyperactivity: motor hyperactivity (shaking, jerking extremities), fasciculations, restlessness
    - Cranial nerve dysfunction: opsoclonus (roving eye movements), slurred speech, tongue fasciculations, hypersalivation, upper airway dysfunction, difficulty swallowing
- Other signs: tachycardia, hypertension, vomiting, stridor, hypoxia, respiratory distress, fever
- Anaphylaxis can occur

Diagnostics
- None

Treatment
- ABCDE
- Grade I and II envenomations often managed at home with OTC analgesia (NSAIDs, acetaminophen)
- Grade III and IV envenomations may require management in health care facility
- Securing airway and ensuring oxygenation is primary concern
- Focus is on control of pain and excessive motor activity
  - Oral agents (oxycodone, oral benzodiazepine) may be sufficient for adults
  - Although titration of IV opioids and benzodiazepines is typically necessary
    - Fentanyl: 1-2 mcg/kg IV q30min PRN pain (preferred agent because of minimal histamine release)
    - Midazolam
      - Adult: 2-5 mg IV q10min
      - Pediatric: 0.05-0.2 mg/kg IV q10min
- Vomiting
  - Typically transient and self-limited
  - Can be treated with anti-emetics

- Hypersalivation
  - Atropine: effectiveness not substantiated
    - Pediatric: 0.05-0.1 mg/kg (min 0.1 mg) IV × 1 dose
- Antivenom
  - If unavailable, treatment is focused on airway protection and titration of benzodiazepines and opioids
  - Use for Grade III or IV envenomation
  - Centruroides (scorpion) specific F(ab')2 equine antivenom
    - 3 vials IV over 10 min
    - Additional 1 vial as needed q30-60min for symptom control
    - If 5 vials given without improvement or resolution consider alternative diagnosis
  - Contraindications: Known hypersensitivity to Centruroides specific F(ab')2 or horses
  - Monitor for signs of hypersensitivity and be prepared to treat (epinephrine, diphenhydramine, corticosteroids)

Disposition
- Discharge Grade III or Grade IV
  - After treatment with antivenom
  - Upon resolution of signs and symptoms
  - Normal vital signs
  - Ambulating without difficulty
- Admit
  - Grade III-IV treated with supportive care requiring titration of IV opioids and analgesia
  - Patients who required intubation for airway protection
  - Complications (aspiration, etc.)

SNAKES

Elapidae

Sources
- Eastern Coral

  PEARL. "Red on yellow kills a fellow…" rhyme only works for North American Coral snakes and is not 100% effective

  - A black snout also distinguishes from the non-venomous king snake
  - Coral snakes may latch on or chew to deliver venom
- Texas Coral

- Sonoran Coral (does not produce clinically dangerous envenomation syndrome)
- Non-native elapid (cobras, mambas, etc.) envenomations in U.S. may occur in setting of exotic pets or zoos
  - Management of non-native elapids is not covered here

Mechanism of Action
- Venom is α-neurotoxins
- Post synaptic neuro-muscular junction blockade

Clinical Manifestations
- Minimal local symptoms
- CNS
  - Paresthesia
  - Dysarthria
  - Ptosis
  - Dysphagia
  - Stridor
  - Diplopia
  - Fasciculations
  - Muscle weakness
  - Paralysis

Diagnostics
- As clinically indicated

Treatment
- ABCDE
- Respiratory support
- Antivenom
  - Systemic toxicity
  - Can decrease length or need at all for mechanical ventilation
  - Eastern Coral
    - Confirmed Eastern Coral with minimal to no symptoms: 3 vials
    - Confirmed Eastern Coral with moderate to severe or systemic symptoms: 5 vials

Disposition

PEARL. Admit all patients even if asymptomatic for frequent neurologic examinations (onset of symptoms up to 13 hrs after envenomation has been reported)

Viperidae (Pit Viper)

Sources
- Majority of U.S. venomous snake bites
- *Crotalinae: Crotalus* (rattlesnakes)
- *Agkistrodon* (copperhead and cottonmouth)
- *Sistrurus* (Massasauga and Pygmy Rattlesnake)

Mechanism of Action
- Venom is a complex mixture of metalloproteinases, phospholipases A_2, hyaluronidase, serine proteases, c-type-lectinlike proteins, disintegrins
- Myotoxic
  - Multiple cytotoxic and proteolytic compounds
- Hemotoxic
  - Consumption of coagulation factors and platelet dysfunction; pro-coagulant and anti-coagulant effects
- Neurotoxic (less common and only in some species)
  - Act at NMJ preventing acetylcholine release
  - Mojave, South Pacific

Clinical Manifestations
- Local tissue injury
  - Severe pain
  - Edema
  - Ecchymosis
  - Hemorrhagic bullae

  PEARL. Consider early intubation in patients with bites to the face or neck area

- Heme
  - Prolonged PT
  - Thrombocytopenia
  - Hypofibrinogenemia
- Systemic effects
  - N/V/D
  - Hypotension
  - Airway edema
  - Systemic toxicity can be difficult to distinguish from anaphylaxis
  - CV collapse
  - Rhabdomyolysis
    - Canebrake
    - Southern Pacific
    - Mojave

- Myokymia/Fasciculations
  - Increased risk of respiratory compromise if present in the upper extremities and torso
  - Mojave, Timber, Southern Pacific rattlesnakes
- Weakness/respiratory failure
  - Mojave

Diagnostics

- PT
- Fibrinogen
- CBC
- CPK in appropriate species

Treatment

- ABCDE
- Antivenom as indicated by diagram on next page
- Epinephrine and IVF for systemic toxicity or suspected anaphylaxis (in addition to AV)
- Elevate and immobilize affected extremity
- Update tetanus

PEARL. Prophylactic antibiotics are not indicated

Disposition

- Observe 8-12 hrs (longer time period for lower extremity bites)
- Discharge "dry bite" after 8 hrs observation and 2 sets of normal labs with no or minimal local signs
- Admit all envenomations and those requiring antivenom treatment

Emergency Department and Hospital Management of Pit Viper Snakebite
Includes: Rattlesnakes, Copperheads, and Cottonmouths (Water Moccasins)

Assess Patient
- Mark leading edge of swelling and tenderness every 15-30 minutes Immobilize and elevate extremity
- Treat pain (IV opioids preferred)
- Obtain initial lab studies (protime, Hgb, platelets, fibrinogen) Update tetanus
- Contact poison control center (1-800-222-1222)

Check for Signs of Envenomation
- Swelling, tenderness, redness, ecchymosis, or blebs at the bite site, *or*
- Elevated protime; decreased fibrinogen or platelets, *or*
- Systemic signs, such as hypotension, bleeding beyond the puncture site, refractory vomiting, diarrhea, angioedema, neurotoxicity

If present continue to Box 3; if none present continue to Box 9

Check for Indications for Antivenom
- Swelling that is more than minimal and that is progressing, *or*
- Elevated protime; decreased fibrinogen or platelets, or
- Any systemic signs

If present continue to Box 4; if none present continue to Box 10

Administer Antivenom
- Establish IV access and give IV fluids
- Pediatric antivenom dose = adult dose
- Mix 4-6 vials of crotaline Fab antivenom (CroFab®) in 250 mL NSS and infuse IV over 1 hr
  — For patients in shock or with serious active bleeding
    • Increase initial dose of antivenom to 8-12 vials
    • Call physician expert (*see box 12*)
- Initiate first dose of antivenom in ED or ICU
  — For suspected adverse reaction: hold infusion, treat accordingly, and call physician-expert
- Re-examine patient for treatment response within 1 hr of completion of antivenom infusion

Continue to Box 5 next page

Determine if Initial Control of Envenomation has been Achieved — 5
- Swelling and tenderness not progressing
- Protime, fibrinogen, and platelets normal or clearly improving
- Clinically stable (not hypotensive, etc.)
- Neurotoxicity resolved or clearly improving

If 'Yes' continue to Box 6; if 'No' continue to Box 11

Monitor Patient — 6
- Perform serial examinations
- Maintenance antivenom therapy may be indicated
  - *Read Box 13 (Maintenance Antivenom Therapy)*
- Observe patient 18-24 hrs after initial control for progression of any venom effect
- Follow-up labs 6-12 hrs after initial control and prior to discharge

If patient develops new or worsening signs of envenomation, administer additional antivenom per Box 4

Determine if Patient Meets Discharge Criteria — 7
- No progression of any venom effect during the specified observation period
- No unfavorable laboratory trends in protime, fibrinogen, or platelets

See Post-Discharge Planning (Box 14) — 8

Apparent Dry Bite/No Bite — 9
- Do not administer antivenom
- Observe patient ≥ 8 hrs
- Repeat labs prior to discharge

If patient develops signs of envenomation, return to Box 2; if not, proceed to Box 7

Apparent Minor Envenomation — 10
- Do not administer antivenom
- Observe patient 12-24 hrs
- Repeat labs at 4-6 hrs and prior to discharge

If patient develops progression of any signs of envenomation, return to Box 3; if not proceed to Box 7

Repeat antivenom until initial control is achieved — 11
If initial control is not achieved after 2 doses of antivenom (Box 4), call physician expert (see Box 12, next page)

When to Call a Physician-Expert

Direct consultation with a physician-expert is recommended in certain high-risk clinical situations:

- **Life-threatening envenomation**
  Shock
  Serious active bleeding
  Facial or airway swelling
- **Hard to control envenomation**
  Envenomation that requires more than 2 doses of antivenom for initial control
- **Recurrence or delayed-onset of venom effects**
  Worsening swelling or abnormal labs (protime, fibrinogen, platelets, or hemoglobin) on follow-up visits
- **Allergic reactions to antivenom**
- **If transfusion is considered**
- **Uncommon clinical situations**
  Bites to the head and neck
  Rhabdomyolysis
  Suspected compartment syndrome
  Venom-induced hives and angioedema
- **Complicated wound issues**

If no local expert is available, a physician-expert can be reached through a certified poison center (1-800-222-1222) or the antivenom manufacturer's line (1-877-377-3784).

Maintenance Antivenom Therapy

- Maintenance therapy is additional antivenom given after initial control to prevent recurrence of limb swelling
  - Maintenance therapy is 2 vials of antivenom q6hrs × 3 (given 6, 12, and 18 hrs after initial control)
- Maintenance therapy may not be indicated in certain situations, such as
  - Minor envenomations
  - Facilities where close observation by a physician-expert is available.
- Follow local protocol or contact a poison center or physician-expert for advice.

Post-Discharge Planning

- Instruct patient to return for
  - Worsening swelling that is not relieved by elevation
  - Abnormal bleeding (gums, easy bruising, melena, etc.)
- Instruct patient where to seek care if symptoms of serum sickness (fever, rash, muscle/joint pains) develop
- Bleeding precautions (no contact sports, elective surgery or dental work, etc.) for 2 weeks in patients with
  - Rattlesnake envenomation
  - Abnormal protime, fibrinogen, or platelet count at any time
- Follow-up visits:
  - Antivenom not given:
    - PRN only

  Antivenom given:
    - Copperhead victims: PRN only
    - Other snakes: Follow up with labs (protime, fibrinogen, platelets, hemoglobin) twice (2-3 days and 5-7 days), then PRN

Treatments to Avoid in Pit Viper Snakebite

- Cutting and/or suctioning of the wound
- Ice
- NSAIDs
- Prophylactic antibiotics
- Prophylactic fasciotomy
- Routine use of blood products
- Shock therapy (electricity)
- Steroids (except for allergic phenomena)
- Tourniquets

Source: Lavonas et al. *BMC Emergency Medicine*. 2011; 11:2 http://www.biomedcentral.com/1471-227X/11/2 (3 February 2011)

Notes

- **All treatment recommendations in this algorithm refer to crotalidae polyvalent immune Fab (ovine) (CroFab®).**
- This worksheet represents general advice from a panel of U.S. snakebite experts convened in May, 2010. No algorithm can anticipate all clinical situations. Other valid approaches exist, and deviations from this worksheet based on individual patient needs, local resources, local treatment guidelines, and patient preferences are expected. **This document is not intended to represent a standard of care.** For more information, please see the accompanying manuscript, available at www.biomedcentral.com.

Heavy Metals

ARSENIC/ARSINE

Sources
- Inorganic (Trivalent and Pentavalent Arsenic)
  - Groundwater and soil
  - Occupational/manufacturing
  - Contaminated xenobiotics/foodstuff
  - Insecticide/pesticide
  - Medicinal (arsenic trioxide for chemotherapy)
- Organic (Arsenobetaine)
  - Seafood
- Arsine gas

Toxic Dose
- Inorganic: Ingestion 100-300 mg trivalent arsenic can be fatal
- Organic: Generally nontoxic
- Arsine gas
  - 25-50 ppm: Lethal after 30 min
  - 3-10 ppm: Exposure may induce symptoms in hours

Mechanism of Action
- Inorganic
  - Binds sulfhydryl groups for critical enzymes
  - Disrupts oxidative phosphorylation causing tissue hypoxia
  - Blocks of cardiac potassium channels
- Arsine gas (liberated when organic arsenic reacts with acid)
  - Binds to erythrocytes and exerts oxidative stress

Clinical Manifestations
- CNS
  - Encephalopathy
  - Weakness
  - Peripheral neuropathy
- CV
  - QT prolongation
  - Ventricular dysrhythmias including torsades de pointes
  - Shock

- Derm (typically after chronic exposure)
  - Alopecia
  - Melanosis and hyperkeratosis
  - Hyperpigmentation
  - Mees' lines
- GI
  - Metallic/garlic taste in mouth
  - Dysphagia
  - Vomiting, diarrhea, and abdominal pain
  - Hematemesis
- Heme
  - Pancytopenia (chronic)
- Renal
  - Renal failure
- Pulmonary
  - Acute lung injury
  - Respiratory failure
- Carcinogenic
- Arsine gas

  PEARL. Hemolysis, bronze-colored skin, hematuria

Diagnostics

- Urine arsenic typically reported as a combination of organic (nontoxic) and inorganic, therefore speciation of urine arsenic will be most accurate
  - Urine spot: > 50 mcg/dL warrants further investigation
- 4 hr urine: < 50 mcg/L normal
- Whole blood arsenic concentration
- BMP
- EKG
- CBC
- CXR
- Toxic Concentrations
  - Inorganic arsenic (trivalent or pentavalent arsenic)
    - Normal whole blood < 5 mcg/L
  - Organic arsenic (arsenobetaine)
    - Frequent cause of elevated arsenic concentrations but non toxic

Treatment
- ABCDE
- Decontamination of skin and clothing
- Chelation therapy
  - Severe systemic toxicity
  - Dose not established
  - Dimercaprol
    - 3.0 mg/kg/dose IM q4hrs for 2 days, then q12hrs for 7-10 days
    - Avoid acidic urine
  - DMSA
    - Adult
      - 10 mg/kg TID for first 5 days
      - Then 10 mg/kg bid for next 14 days
    - Children
      - 350 mg/m^2 TID for the first 5 days
      - Then 350 mg/m^2 BID for the next 14 days
- Arsine hemolysis
  - Exchange transfusion
  - Plasmophoresis
  - HD

Disposition
- Admit
  - Severe, persistent, or worsening signs and symptoms or those requiring chelation treatment

IRON

Sources
- Prenatal vitamins
- Iron supplements

Toxic Dose
- Low toxicity: < 20 mg/kg elemental iron
- Moderate toxicity: 20-60 mg/kg elemental iron
- Severe toxicity: > 60 mg/kg elemental iron

Mechanism of Action
- Free radical formation leading to oxidative damage to the GI mucosa
- Free iron inhibits thrombin leading to coagulopathy
- Inhibits oxidative phosphorylation

Clinical Manifestations
- Up to 6 hrs after ingestion
  - Abdominal pain
  - N/V/D

  PEARL. If no symptoms in the first 6 hrs, unlikely to develop toxicity

- 6-24 hrs
  - GI symptoms abate
  - Progressive toxicity and organ damage ensue
  - Metabolic acidosis
- 12-24 hrs
  - Hemodynamic compromise
  - Coagulopathy
  - Metabolic acidosis
- Within 48 hrs
  - Hepatotoxicity
- 3-6 weeks after ingestion
  - Potential GI strictures

Diagnostics
- Serum iron concentration
  - Measure at 4 hrs post ingestion and serially. (Serial concentration needed because peak can be delayed)
  - 300-500 mcg/dL typically associated with significant GI symptoms
  - > 500 mcg/dL typically associated with systemic symptoms

  PEARL. Must be correlated with clinical findings to determine toxicity

- BMP
- Abdominal radiograph
  - May not detect liquid preparations or dissolved
  - May be positive in the absence of clinical manifestations

Treatment
- ABCDE
- Whole bowel irrigation
  - Consider if large amount of iron on abdominal radiograph
- Severe iron poisoning is treated with the chelator deferoxamine
  - **Dosing:** 5 mg/kg/hr, increasing if tolerated to 15 mg/kg/hr; max 6 g/day
  - **Indications**
    - Signs and symptoms with serum iron concentration > 500 mcg/dL
    - Significant clinical manifestations regardless of concentration
      - Hypotension
      - Lethargy
      - Coma

- ♦ Shock
- ♦ Metabolic acidosis
— Adverse effects of deferoxamine
  - ♦ Hypotension
  - ♦ ARDS
  - ♦ Yersinia enterocolitica infection

Disposition
- Observe minimum 6 hrs
- Admit severe, persistent, or worsening signs and symptoms or those requiring chelation treatment

LEAD

Sources
- Lead-based paints and solder
- Occupational (welding, battery manufacture, mining)
- Bullets
- Ceramics
- Moonshine
- Contaminated food, water, soil, and complementary remedies

Toxic Dose
- Not naturally found in the body; even concentrations < 10 mc/dL potentially harmful in children

Mechanism of Action
- Inhibits ferrochelatase and inhibits delta ALA dehydratase, resulting in reduction of heme
- Mimics Ca^{2+}
  — Disrupts cell signaling (disrupts activation of protein kinase C), leading to the neurotoxic effects
- Interferes with collagen synthesis and vascular permeability of blood-brain barrier

Clinical Manifestations
- ACUTE
  — Abdominal pain
  — N/V
  — HTN
  — Headache
  — Encephalopathy
  — Increased ICP

- CHRONIC
  - The most concerning and widely studied clinical effect of chronic lead exposure is neurocognitive developmental delay in children, which is thought to potentially occur even at BLL < 10 mcg/dL
  - Following signs and symptoms typically seen with these ranges of BLL:
    - Pediatric
      - Up to 50 mcg/dL: Asymptomatic, but concern for decrement on cognitive development, growth
      - 50-70 mcg/dL: Mild to moderate toxicity, abdominal pain, vomiting, anorexia, irritability
      - 70-100 mcg/dL: Severe toxicity, encephalopathy, anemia
    - Adult
      - 20-69 mcg/dL: Asymptomatic, but may have HTN, renal insufficiency, decreased bone density
      - 70-100 mcg/dL: Moderate toxicity, memory loss, neuropathy, abdominal pain, nephropathy, mild anemia
      - > 100 mcg/dL: Severe toxicity, encephalopathy, anemia, nephropathy

Diagnostics
- Whole blood lead level (BLL)
  - Toxic concentration: > 70-100 mcg/dL typically associated with lead encephalopathy
- Zinc or free protoporphyrin may help differentiate acute vs. chronic
- CBC
- BMP
- Radiographs: Suspected or known ingestions or retained bullet fragments

Treatment
- ABCDE
- Terminate exposure
  - If suspected household exposure, must contact local health department for remediation
- Decontamination
  - Consider whole bowel irrigation for ingested lead such as paint chips on abdominal radiograph
- Chelation therapy
  - All patients with lead encephalopathy
  - All patients who are symptomatic with BLL > 70 mcg/dL
  - Pediatric patients with BLL > 45 mcg/dL even if asymptomatic
  - Decisions regarding chelation therapy often case-based

- **Chelation Therapy Details**
  - DMSA (succimer) in patients without encephalopathy
  - Adult and pediatric: 10 mg/kg PO q8 hours × 5 days; then q12hrs × 14 days (max 500 mg/dose)
- Acute Lead Encephalopathy
  - FIRST administer dimercaprol—4 mg/kg (75 mg/m^2) deep IM given alone in 1st dose and then q4hrs in combination with calcium EDTA administered at separate site
    - Calcium EDTA—1500 mg/m^2/day as continuous infusion starting 4 hrs after initial dose of dimercaprol, max 3 g/day
      - Adjust dose in patients with impaired renal function

Disposition

- Admit
  - Symptomatic lead poisoning, particularly concern for lead encephalopathy
  - Severe, persistent, or worsening signs and symptoms or those requiring chelation treatment

  PEARL. Consider admitting children to allow for home remediation if social situation difficult

MERCURY

Sources

- Elemental: Thermometers/barometers, tissue fixatives
- Inorganic: Dyes, laboratory reagents, tanneries, calomel
- Organic: Laboratory reagents, wood preservatives, pharmaceuticals, seafood

Toxic Dose

- Elemental: Airborne exposure of 10 mg/m^3 IDLH
- Inorganic: Lethal oral dose 1-4 g
- Organic: Ingestion 10-60 mg/kg may be fatal

Mechanism of Action

- Interruption of microtubule formation
- Changing intracellular calcium balance and membrane potential
- Oxidative stress
- Disturbing enzyme and protein function
- Inhaled mercury vapor (elemental) or ingested ethyl mercury (organic) undergo conversion to inorganic mercury endogenously

Clinical Manifestations
- **Elemental mercury** exposure typically via inhalation of mercury vapor but ingestions, vascular, and subcutaneous injections also reported
  - ACUTE
    - Respiratory
      - Cough
      - Shortness of breath
      - ARDS
  - CHRONIC
    - Erethism
      - "Mad Hatter"
      - Tremor
      - Gingivostomatitis
      - Neuropsychiatric changes
- **Inorganic mercury** (mercuric chloride)
  - ACUTE
    - GI
      - N/V/D
      - Metallic taste
    - Renal
      - Renal dysfunction
  - CHRONIC

    PEARL. Acrodynia (aka "Pink's Disease", erythema, pain and swelling in digits, photophobia, irritability, sweatiness, tremors)
      - Erethism
- **Organic mercury** (methyl mercury)
  - CNS
    - Delayed
    - Paresthesias of hands and feet
    - Ataxia
    - Encephalopathy
  - Teratogen
    - Developmental delay, spasticity, deafness, blindness, seizures

Diagnostics
- Urine spot concentration if acute poisoning suspected
  - Normal concentration in urine: < 20 mcg/L
- 24 hr urine concentration confirmatory
- Whole blood concentration for methyl mercury (organic)
  - Normal concentration in blood: < 10.0 mcg/L
- BMP

Treatment
- ABCDE
- Chelation therapy only effective for mercury vapor and inorganic mercury (not used for methyl mercury or ethyl mercury)
  - Severe systemic toxicity
  - Dimercaprol (3 steps)
    - 5 mg/kg IM once
    - 2.5 mg/kg IM every 8-12 hrs for 1 day
    - Then 2.5 mg/kg IM every 12-24 hrs for 7 days
  - DMSA
    - Adult
      - 10 mg/kg TID for first 5 days
      - Then 10 mg/kg bid for next 14 days
    - Children
      - 350 mg/m2 TID for the first 5 days
      - Then 350 mg/m2 BID for the next 14 days
  - Penicillamine (serious adverse effects limit the use of this chelator)
    - Adults
      - 250 mg QID PO for 1-2 weeks
    - Children
      - 20-30 mg/kg/daily in 4 divided doses, max 250/dose

Disposition
- Admit severe, persistent, or worsening signs and symptoms or those requiring chelation treatment

METAL FUME FEVER

Source
- Welding/smelting galvanized metal, typically steel that contains zinc

Toxic Dose
- Inhalation: 77-600 mg Zn/m^3

Mechanism of Action
- Proinflammatory cytokine release
- Neutrophil activation
- Oxygen radical formation from zinc (most common), chrome, nickel, copper, manganese

Clinical Manifestations
- 4-10 hrs after exposure to metal fumes
  - Fever
  - Chills
  - Myalgias
  - Headache
  - Malaise
  - Cough, chest pain, dyspnea

PEARL. Tachyphylaxis occurs; relief of symptoms during days off and return of symptoms when return to work

Diagnostics
- No specific test
- CXR typically normal

Treatment
- ABCDE
- NSAIDs
- Bronchodilator
- Personal protection equipment at workplace

Disposition
- Observe minimum 6 hrs
- Admit severe, persistent, or worsening signs and symptoms

THALLIUM

Sources
- Salts
- Occupational (smelting)
- Rodenticides
- Nuclear Medicine testing

Toxic Dose
- 6-40 mg/kg: Fatalities reported

Mechanism of Action
- Thallium is treated like potassium in the body because of its biochemical similarity
- Interferes with glycolysis, Kreb's cycle, and oxidative phosphorylation
- Bind sulfhydryl groups on the mitochondrial membrane to interrupt the activity of sodium–potassium ATPase

Clinical Manifestations
- CNS

    PEARL. Ascending neuropathy (extremely painful) days after exposure
    - Motor weakness
    - Encephalopathy
    - Seizures
    - Coma
    - Optic neuritis
- CV
    - Tachycardia and hypertension
- Derm
    - Alopecia (delayed 1-2 weeks)
    - Mees' lines
- GI
    - N/V
    - Abdominal pain

Diagnostics
- Blood thallium concentration
- 24 hr urine: < 5 mcg/L normal
- BMP
- CBC
- EKG
- Consider abdominal radiographs if ingested

Treatment
- ABCDE
- Consider multi-dose activated charcoal because of enterohepatic recirculation

    PEARL. Prussian blue 250 mg/kg/day PO or NG divided over 3-4 doses
    - Systemic toxicity

Disposition
- Admit severe, persistent, or worsening signs and symptoms or those requiring chelation treatment

Hemoglobinopathies

CARBON MONOXIDE

Sources
- Colorless, odorless gas
- Incomplete combustion of carbonaceous fuels
  - Charcoal
  - Wood
  - Natural gas
  - Propane
- Structure fires
- Improperly vented stoves
- Portable heaters
- Automobile exhaust

PEARL. Methylene chloride, found in degreasers and solvents, metabolized to CO in delayed fashion

Toxic Dose
- 1200 ppm IDLH
- Duration of exposure also important

Mechanism of Action
- ACUTE toxicity
  - CO binds hemoglobin with 250X greater affinity than O_2
  - Greater affinity than O_2 for cardiac myoglobin causing myocardial depression
  - Creates functional anemia and left shift of oxyhemoglobin dissociation curve
  - CO increases nitric oxide and activates cGMP resulting in vasodilation and hypotension
  - Inhibits cytochrome oxidase c
- Possible delayed cognitive sequelae
  - Interferes with cellular respiration leading to ischemic reperfusion injury
  - Causes immune cascade and delayed lipid peroxidation

Clinical Manifestations
- ACUTE toxicity
  - Most common
    - Headache
    - N/V
    - Dizziness

- CV
  - Tachycardia
  - Hypotension
  - Premature ventricular contraction
  - Angina
  - Elevated troponin
  - Cardiac arrest
- CNS
  - Ataxia
  - Syncope/loss of consciousness
  - Seizure
  - Coma
- Pulmonary
  - Dyspnea/SOB
  - Tachypnea/increased respiratory rate

PEARL. "Cherry red" tissues are not seen until very late in clinical course or post-mortem

- Delayed neurologic sequelae
  - Dementia
  - Parkinsonism
  - Chorea
  - Psychosis
  - Apraxia
  - Agnosia
  - Neuropathy

PEARL. Risk factors for delayed neurologic sequelae include loss of consciousness, hypotension, and older age

Diagnostics

- SpO_2
  - Falsely reads normal to mildly low
- Pulse CO-oximeter
- CO Hgb
  - May be performed on either arterial or venous blood
  - 0-5% normal in nonsmokers, > 5% abnormal
  - 6-10% normal in smokers, > 10% abnormal

PEARL. Concentration may NOT be predictive of symptom severity

- ABG/VBG
- Troponin
- CPK

- EKG
- Lactate
- CXR
- Head CT (to evaluate for alternative diagnosis acutely)

Treatment
- ABCDE
- Removal from source
- 100% O_2, either via non-rebreather or intubation and mechanical ventilation, depending on clinical severity

PEARL. Consider concomitant CN poisoning in fire victims and recommend avoiding sodium nitrite administration in these patients

- Supportive care remains primary focus, fluid resuscitation, vasopressors and inotropes, ACLS protocol for dysrhythmias
- Hyperbaric oxygen remains controversial; benefit remains unproven
  - Potential or cited indications
    - Altered level of consciousness
    - Coma
    - Seizure
    - Abnormal cerebellar or focal neurologic exam
    - CO Hgb > 25%
    - CO Hgb > 10% in pregnant woman

PEARL. Must identify source of CO poisoning to ensure patient does not return to unsafe environment

Disposition
- Admit severe, persistent, or worsening signs and symptoms or those requiring hyperbaric oxygen therapy

METHEMOGLOBINEMIA

Sources
- Congenital (eg, deficiency of NADH methemoglobin reductase, also known as cytochrome b5 reductase; hemoglobin M)
- Infection
  - Neonates
- Medications
  - Amyl nitrite
  - Benzocaine
  - Lidocaine
  - Prilocaine
  - Dapsone

- Nitric oxide
- Nitroprusside
- Nitroglycerin
- Phenazopyridine
- Quinones
- Sulfonamides
- Xenobiotics
  - Nitrites/nitrates
  - Aniline dye
  - Chlorobenzene
  - Naphthalene
  - Trinitrotoluene

Toxic Dose
- Highly variable and dependent upon toxin and route of exposure

Mechanism of Action
- Medications and xenobiotics oxidize iron in hemoglobin from ferrous [Fe^{2+} to ferric (Fe^{3+})] state, creating methemoglobin
- Methemoglobin unable to carry oxygen
  - Functional anemia
  - Oxygen-hemoglobin dissociation curve shifted to left

Clinical Manifestations
- 10-20%
  - Cyanosis (assuming a normal hemoglobin concentration)
- 20-50%
  - Dizziness
  - Fatigue
  - Headache
  - Exertional dyspnea
  - Anxiety
- 50%
  - Lethargy
  - Stupor
  - Metabolic acidosis
  - Dysrhythmias
- \> 70%
  - Lethal

PEARL. Expect more severe symptoms in patients with underlying anemia, CHF, COPD, pneumonia

Diagnostics

PEARL. "Chocolate brown blood"

PEARL. Cyanosis and abnormal pulse oximeter (~85%) unresponsive to O_2

- ABG/VBG
- Venous/arterial MetHb concentration via co-oximetry
- EKG
- CMP
- CBC

Treatment
- Methylene blue
  - \> 30% MetHb and symptomatic
  - 1-2 mg/kg IV over 5 min (0.1-0.2 mL/kg of 1% solution)
  - Repeat dose if symptoms persist or MetHb > 30%

  PEARL. Methylene blue can interfere with pulse-oximetry, resulting in decreased oxygen saturation on monitor

  - G6PD deficiency
    - Methylene blue contraindicated if known G6PD deficiency (low NADPH production impairs NADPH methemoglobin reductase function so methylene blue would have minimal effect) and may precipitate hemolysis
    - Consider exchange transfusion or HBO
  - NADPH MetHb reductase deficiency
    - Neonates or congenital
    - May not respond fully to methylene blue
  - Dapsone and aniline
    - May require repeat methylene blue administration or continuous infusion
    - Consider cimetidine 400 mg TID (cyp450 inhibitor)
      - Dapsone

Disposition
- Admit severe, persistent, or worsening signs and symptoms or those requiring antidotal treatment for refractory or long-acting oxidizing agent

Mushrooms

MUSHROOMS (*A. PHALLOIDES, GYROMITRA, A. MUSCARIA, PSILOCYBE, COPRINUS, CLITOCYBE/INOCYBE, C. ORELLANUS, T. EQUESTRE, A. SMITHIANA*)

Sources
- Fruiting body of a fungus
- Lack chlorophyll
- Found throughout most of North America

Toxic Dose
- Amatoxin: Minimal lethal dose 0.1 mg/kg (1 *Amanita phalloides* can contain 10-15 mg)
- *Gyromitra*: Estimated lethal dose 20-50 mg/kg adult; 10-30 mg/kg children

Mechanisms of Action
- Inhibits RNA polymerase II-> DNA transcription arrest
  - *Amanita phalloides* ("death cap"), *Lepiota* spp., *Galerina* spp.
  - α-Amanitin (amatoxin)
  - Hepatotoxicity
  - Majority of fatalities (> 90%)
- Pyridoxine inhibition
  - *Gyromitra* spp. ("false morel")
  - Seizures
- GABA/glutamate agonism
  - *Amanita muscaria*
  - Muscimol
    - $GABA_A$ agonist
    - Coma
  - Ibotenic acid
    - Glutamate agonism
    - Seizures
- Serotonergic
  - *Psilocybe* spp.
- Acetaldehyde inhibition
  - *Coprinus* spp.
  - 1-Aminocyclopropanol

- Cholinergic (peripheral)
  - *Clitocybe/Inocybe* spp.
  - Muscarine

Clinical Manifestations
- Several toxidromes associated with different species
- < 6 hrs from ingestion

> **PEARL.** Presentations with symptoms occurring < **6 hrs from ingestion** more likely benign, self-limiting

  - *Chlorophyllum molybdites* (common lawn mushroom)
    - N/V/D
  - *Psilocybe* spp.
    - Hallucinogenic effects
  - *Amanita muscaria*
    - Seizures
    - Coma
  - *Clitocybe, Inocybe* spp.
    - Cholinergic
  - *Coprinus* spp.
    - Disulfiram effect
- > 6 hrs from ingestion

> **PEARL.** Onset of symptoms > **6 hrs from ingestion** portends a more severe toxicity

  - Commonly starts with GI symptoms: nausea, vomiting
  - *Amanita phalloides*
    - GI signs and symptoms 6-24 hrs after ingestion with apparent clinical improvement for 24 hrs before hepatic injury progresses to either acute hepatic failure or recovery
  - *Gyromitra* spp.
    - Seizure
    - Ataxia
    - Hemolysis
    - Methemoglobinemia (See p. 87)
  - *Cortinarius orellanus*
    - Delayed renal failure (1-6 days)
  - *Tricholoma equestre*
    - Delayed myotoxicity
    - Rhabdomyolysis

> **PEARL.** EXCEPTION: *Amanita smithiana*; early GI symptoms, delayed renal failure

Diagnostics

PEARL. Attempt to obtain mushroom or picture to identify

- BMP
- CBC
- PT/INR
- CPK
- LFT

Treatment

- ABCDE
- Hepatotoxicity (*A. phalloides*)
  - N-acetylcysteine IV dosing
    - Load: 150 mg/kg for 60 min, then 50 mg/kg for 4 hrs, then 100 mg/kg for 16 hrs
    - If on intermittent HD (IHD): double dose during IHD with additional ½ load when IHD > 6 hrs
  - Penicillin
    - Day 1: 1,000,000 U/kg IV
    - Days 2 and 3: 500,000 U/kg IV
  - Silimarin [milk thistle extract]
    - Not approved by FDA, but can be acquired from researchers at clinicaltrials.gov
    - If available should be used alone or with NAC but not penicillin
    - 5 mg/kg IV, followed by 20 mg/kg continuous infusion over 24 hrs
- Nephrotoxicity (*Cortinarius, A. smithiana*)
  - Renal support
  - Hemodialysis
- Rhabdomyolysis (*T. equestre*)
  - IVF
  - Renal support
- Seizures (*Gyromitra* spp.)
  - Diazepam
    - Adult: 5-10 mg IV q5-10min PRN
    - Pediatric: 0.2-0.5 mg/kg IV q5-10min PRN
  - Lorazepam
    - Adult: 2-4 mg IV q10-15min PRN
    - Pediatric: 0.05-0.1 mg/kg IV q10-15min PRN
  - Propofol (if intubated)
    - Continuous infusion of 5 mcg/kg/min titrate (rec. max of 55 mcg/kg/min)

PEARL. If resistant to treatment administer pyridoxine 5 g IV

- Hallucinations
  - Benzodiazepines
  - Haloperidol
    - Adult: 5 mg IV/IM, repeat PRN 10-30 min
- Cholinergic
  - Atropine
    - Adult: 1-2 mg IV slow push, double dose q3-5min until dry
      - Maintenance 10-20% of load IV qh, titrate PRN
    - Pediatric: 0.02 mg/kg (min 0.1 mg) IV. Double the dose if previous does not induce atropinization

Disposition
- Admit
  - Severe, persistent, or worsening signs and symptoms
  - Unclear clinical picture or timing of exposure with concern for possible delayed poisoning

PHARMACOLOGIC AGENTS

ACETAMINOPHEN/PARACETAMOL (APAP)
Source
- OTC and prescription oral analgesics, cough, and cold preparations
- Often in combination with other medications

Toxic Dose
- Adults: acute ingestion of ≥ 150 mg/kg in adults
- Children: acute ingestion 200 mg/kg

Mechanism of Action
- Analgesic/antipyretic: Prevents the formation of prostaglandin H_2 and E_2 via inhibition of cyclooxygenase-2
- Toxicity: APAP is partially metabolized via cytochrome P450 to N-acetyl-p-benzoquinone imine (NAPQI), a toxic reactive metabolite that causes injury when glutathione stores are overwhelmed

Clinical Manifestations
PEARL. Clinical stages may overlap
- Stage I
  - 0-24 hrs after ingestion
  - LFT typically normal
  - Signs/symptoms
    - Primarily asymptomatic
    - N/V
    - Abdominal pain
    - Malaise
- Stage II
  - 24-72 hrs after ingestion
  - Onset of liver injury
  - AST is the most sensitive test (hepatotoxicity defined as AST > 1,000 IUL)
  - Signs/symptoms
    - Asymptomatic
    - Vomiting
    - RUQ pain

- Stage III
  - 72-96 hrs after ingestion
  - Fulminant hepatic failure
  - LFT > 10,000 are common
  - Signs/symptoms
    - Encephalopathy
    - Renal failure
    - Coagulopathy
    - Metabolic acidosis
    - Cerebral edema
    - Death
- Stage IV
  - 4 days-3 weeks after ingestion
  - Recovery phase, complete hepatic regeneration

PEARL. In massive ingestion patients may present early with coma, AG metabolic acidosis, elevated lactate due to NAPQI mitochondrial toxicity

Diagnostics
- APAP concentration

  PEARL. ≥ 150 mcg/mL at 4 hrs from ingestion = potentially toxic

- LFT
- BMP
- Lactate (massive ingestion)
- NH_3 (altered mental status)
- Lipase
- PT/INR

  PEARL. Early mild elevations may be traced to IV NAC or APAP's ability to inhibit gamma-carboxylation of vitamin K dependent factors and not reflective of hepatic injury

Treatment
- GI decontamination
  - Consider activated charcoal in alert patients within 1 hr post ingestion
- N-acetylcysteine (NAC) indications
  - APAP concentration above the treatment line on the nomogram
  - Measurable APAP concentration with unknown time of ingestion
  - Patients with elevated LFT without prior history of LFT abnormalities in setting of suspected overdose
  - Symptomatic patients (vomiting and/or abdominal pain)

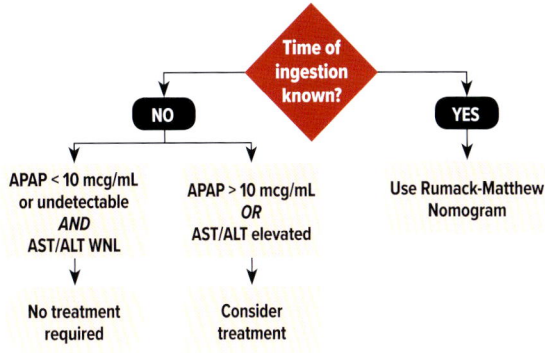

PEARL. IV and oral formulations of NAC are equally efficacious; however, IV route is preferred in patients with hepatic failure, intractable vomiting, or pregnancy.

- NAC IV dosing (21-hr NAC protocol)
  - 150 mg/kg over 60 min
  - Then, 50 mg/kg over 4 hrs (12.5 mg/kg/hr for 4 hrs)
  - Then, 100 mg/kg over 16 hrs (6.25 mg/kg/hr for 16 hrs)
  - May continue at 6.25 mg/kg/hr until discontinuation criteria met
  - IV NAC preparation can result in anaphylactoid reactions (rash, flushing, vomiting, bronchospasm). If anaphylactoid reaction occurs discontinue NAC, administer antihistamine, steroid, and often may resume NAC at slower rate
- NAC oral dosing (72-hr NAC protocol)
  - 140 mg/kg PO loading dose followed by 70 mg/kg PO q4hrs for 17 doses or until discontinuation criteria met
- Dilution recommended to increase palatability
- Continue NAC until recovery, transplant, or death if there is evidence of fulminant hepatic failure
- May discontinue NAC if acetaminophen concentration < 10 mcg/mL and serum AST/ALT and PT are within normal limits or declining and patient clinically improving

- Adjunctive therapy

  > **PEARL.** Hemodialysis should be considered for acute, massive ingestions with severe metabolic acidosis

  — Signs of mitochondrial dysfunction and an APAP concentration > 900 mcg/mL if NAC is administered
  — NAC infusion rate should be at least doubled during intermittent hemodialysis with an additional half loading dose given if hemodialysis exceeds 6 hrs
  — Consider CVVH in cases of fulminant hepatic failure, particularly if metabolic acidosis and/or encephalopathy are present

Disposition

- Admit all who require antidotal treatment

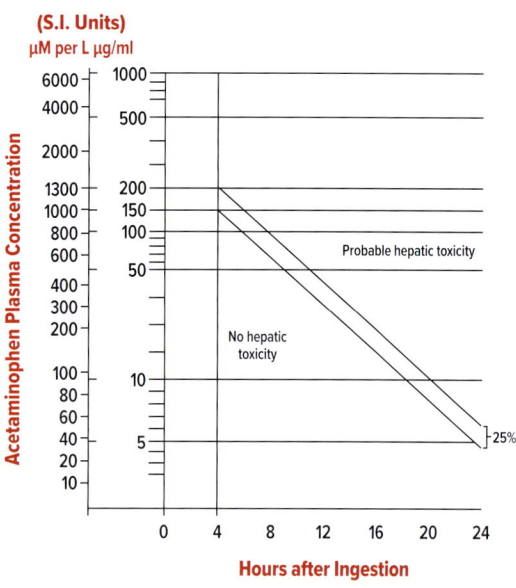

ANESTHETICS

Local

Source
- Injected anesthetics

Toxic Dose
- Exceeding max adult single dose may cause toxicity
  Esters (single 'I')
  — Cocaine
  — Benzocaine
  — Procaine (max adult single dose 600 mg subcutaneous)
  — Tetracaine (max adult single dose 15 mg subcutaneous)
  Amides (2 I's)
  — Lidocaine (max adult single dose 300 mg subcutaneous)
  — Lidocaine with epinephrine (max adult single dose 500 mg subcutaneous)
  — Lidocaine IV
    - Seizures reported with 1.4 mg/kg
    - Cardiac arrest reported after 2.5 mg/kg
  — Mepivacaine (max adult single dose 400 mg subcutaneous)
  — Bupivacaine (max adult single dose 400 mg subcutaneous)
    - Seizures reported with 1.3 mg/kg IV
    - Cardiac arrest reported after 1.6 mg/kg

    PEARL. Sodium benzonatate has structural and clinical similarity

  — Anesthetic toxicity likely to occur:
    - With excessive dosing, repeated therapeutic dosing
    - Highly vascular sites of administration (ie, areas with greater blood flow will have more systemic absorption)
    - Inadvertent intravascular injection, particularly with co-administration of epinephrine
    - Intrathecal pump malfunction or refilling errors

Mechanism of Action
- Reversibly block Na^+ channels
- Inhibit axonal transmission resulting in analgesia

Clinical Manifestations
- Some recommend combining short acting and longer acting local anesthetics to take advantage of their different kinetics
  — In practice, advantage is minimal and toxicity is additive

- < 1% of adverse events are hypersensitivity related (allergic reactions)
  - Esters are responsible for majority of allergic reactions
  - Hypersensitivity reaction from esters commonly caused by reaction to the metabolite para-aminobenzoic acid (PABA)

PEARL. Amides are not metabolized to PABA

  - Multidose preparations of amides may contain the preservative methylparaben, which is similar to PABA
  - Preservative free amides can be used in patients with allergic reactions that are likely caused by methylparaben

PEARL. Cardiac lidocaine is preservative-free and may be safe in patients with hypersensitivity reactions to regular lidocaine

PEARL. If the patient has an allergic reaction to a local anesthetic, a paraben preservative-free drug from the opposite class usually can be administered safely

PEARL. Methemoglobinemia most frequently associated with benzocaine as used for topical anesthesia (eg, bronchoscopy, NG tube placement, teething in infants)

  - In addition to occurring from large doses, can occur because of breaks in the mucosa allowing increased absorption
- Aside from cocaine, all cause peripheral vasodilation
- CNS toxicity normally occurs prior to cardiac toxicity (exception: bupivacaine)
- Mild toxicity
  - Tinnitus
  - Lightheadedness
  - Circumoral numbness
  - Confusion
  - Muscle twitching
  - Psychological symptoms (easily confused with anxiety or effects from co-administered sedatives)
- Severe toxicity
  - Mental status changes
  - Syncope
  - Seizure (acidosis and hypercarbia lower seizure threshold)
  - Dysrhythmias

PEARL. Bupivacaine most cardiotoxic

  - Cardiovascular collapse

Diagnostics
- Serum MetHb concentration
- EKG
- Serum anesthetic concentration (although its utility is limited as may not come back in clinically useful timeframe)

Treatment
- ABCDE
- Local Anesthetic Systemic Toxicity (LAST)
  — Minor symptoms do not require treatment
  — Severe toxicity

  PEARL. Administer lipid emulsion therapy

  - Bolus 1.5 mL/kg IV 20% lipids over 1 min (may repeat once or twice)
  - Continuous infusion 0.25 mL/kg/min. Can double if patient remains hypotensive
  - Continue for 10 min. Recommended upper limit of administration is 10 mL/kg over 30 min

  — Vasopressors for hypotension
  — Standard ACLS for cardiac arrest
  — ECMO
- Seizures
  — Diazepam
    - Adult: 5-10 mg IV q1-2hrs PRN
    - Pediatric: 0.15-0.2 mg/kg IV q5-10min
  — Lorazepam
    - Adult: 2-4 mg IV q1-2hrs PRN
    - Pediatric: 0.1 mg/kg IV q5-10min
  — Phenobarbital
    - 20 mg/kg IV over 20 min
    - High risk for respiratory depression if patient has already received other sedatives
  — Propofol (if intubated)
    - Continuous infusion of 5 mcg/kg/min and titrate to effect
- Methemoglobinemia
  — Methylene blue: 1-2 mg/kg IV
- QRS prolongation
  — IV sodium bicarbonate
    - Bolus: 1-2 mEq/kg IVP over 1-2 min
    - Infusion: 100-150 mEq in 1 L D5W @ 150-200 mL/h (2x maintenance in pediatrics)

Disposition
- Admit
  - Severe, persistent, or worsening signs and symptoms
- Methemoglobinemia: Discharge after treatment and/or resolved, asymptomatic

Nitrous Oxide

Source
- Inhaled anesthetics

Toxic Dose
- **Exceeding max adult single dose may cause toxicity**
  - \> 1000 ppm causes severe toxicity
    - Can be found as the propellant in whipped cream canisters and cartridges Also known as whippets
    - May be abused by adolescents
      > **PEARL.** Abuse potential by health care practitioners, including dentists and dental hygienists

Mechanism of Action
- Stimulate cell synapses resulting in release of inhibitory neurotransmitters and inhibition of excitatory neurotransmitters with variable responses

> **PEARL.** Nitrous oxide abuse causes inactivation of vitamin B12 resulting in impaired DNA and myelin synthesis

- Abuse can result in asphyxiation from oxygen displacement
  - Multiple deceased were discovered with bags over their heads in an attempt to prolong intoxication

Clinical Manifestations
- Commonly abused
- Avoid if pregnant
- CNS
  - Myeloneuropathy with combined subacute degeneration of dorsal columns
  - Producing sensory polyneuropathy with numbness, paresthesias, ataxia, incontinence
- Heme: Bone marrow suppression: leukopenia, megaloblastic erythropoiesis followed by thrombocytopenia.
- Immunologic: Decreased neutrophil chemotaxis

Diagnostics
- CBC
- Vitamin B12 and folate
- Homocysteine and methylmalonic acid concentrations (which should be elevated)
- EMGs for peripheral neuropathy

Treatment
- ABCDE
- Remove exposure
- Supportive respiratory care
- Sensorimotor polyneuropathy
  - Coasting may occur with transient worsening of symptoms after cessation
  - Vitamin B12 and methionine supplementation (limited evidence)

Disposition
- Admit severe, persistent, or worsening signs and symptoms

ANTIDYSRHYTHMICS

Type I

Sources: Three Vaughan-Williams Classes
- Class IA (procainamide, quinidine, disopyramide)
  - Block both Na^+ and K^+ channels
    - K^+ channel blocking prolongs repolarization and refractory period, resulting in prolonged QT interval
    - Na^+ channel blocking slows depolarization, resulting in widened QRS duration
- Class IB (lidocaine, tocainide, mexiletine, moricizine, phenytoin)
  - High affinity for the inactivated Na^+ channel (during depolarization, early repolarization, and ischemia)
  - Binding to Na^+ channel while in its inactivated form is brief
  - Almost no binding during repolarization
  - At therapeutic doses, there is no prolongation of the QRS
  - No effect on myocardial K^+ channel
  - No QT prolongation

- Type 1C (flecainide and propafenone)
  - High affinity for activated Na⁺ channel
  - Binding to Na⁺ channel is prolonged, can persist into next cardiac cycle
  - Prolongs QRS complex
  - Also have calcium and potassium channel blocking properties

Toxic Doses
- Narrow therapeutic index
- Doses 2 times therapeutic may cause toxicity (exception: amiodarone is well-tolerated, even in large doses)

Mechanism of Action
- Medications of all 3 classes bind to voltage-gated fast inward Na⁺ channels
  - Prolonging recovery to resting state
  - Preventing depolarization by additional electrical impulses
- Type IA and IC agents also block K⁺ efflux channels
  - Prolonging repolarization

Clinical Manifestations

PEARL. Toxicity may be seen not only in acute overdose, but also in typical use, medication errors, and therapeutic misadventure

- Type IA
  - Procainamide
    - ACUTE
      - Toxicity may occur when intravenous administration is too rapid
      - Hypotension
      - QRS prolongation
      - Ventricular dysrhythmias
      - Prolonged QT interval
      - Polymorphic VT
    - CHRONIC
      - Long-term use can cause development of antinuclear antibodies and drug-induced lupus
  - Quinidine
    - QRS and QT prolongation with associated ventricular dysrhythmias including torsades de pointes
    - Hypoglycemia—pancreatic K⁺ channel blockade results in increased insulin release
    - Cinchonism—abdominal pain, tinnitus, and delirium

- Disopyramide
  - Congestive heart failure because of negative ionotropic effects of Ca^{2+} channel blockade
  - Anticholinergic toxidrome
  - Hypoglycemia (similar mechanism to quinidine)
- Type IB
  - Lidocaine
    - CNS toxicity—occurs first because of rapid CNS entry
      - Paresthesias
      - Seizures
      - Altered mental status
    - CV toxicity—occurs shortly after CNS toxicity
      - SA/AV nodal depression
      - AV block
      - Sinus arrest possible
      - Can progress to cardiac arrest
  - Mexiletine
    - Similar structure, function, and toxicity as lidocaine
- Type IC
  - Flecainide
    - Most common toxic effect is dysrhythmia, even at therapeutic dose
    - Characteristically causes moderate to marked QRS and PR prolongation with mild QT prolongation
    - Hypotension
    - Bradycardia
    - AV block
    - Ventricular dysrhythmias
  - Propafenone
    - Toxicity manifests as CHF (from β and Ca^{2+} channel blockade effect)
    - Ventricular dysrhythmias
    - Bradycardia

Diagnostics

- Serum concentration available but results likely not timely enough to guide treatment

Treatment

- ABCDE
- GI decontamination
  - Can consider activated charcoal/gastric lavage/whole bowel irrigation especially in large intentional extended release ingestion
  - Must weigh risk:benefit as improved clinical outcome is not substantiated

- QRS prolongation
  - IV sodium bicarbonate
    - Bolus: 1-2 mEq/kg IVP over 1-2 min
    - Infusion: 100-150 mEq in 1 L D5W @ 150-200 mL/h (or roughly 2x maintenance)
  - Titrate until QRS narrows. Monitor serum pH to maximum of 7.55
  - Consider 3% saline if sodium bicarbonate ineffective
    - 50-100 mL IV
- Polymorphic VT (torsades de pointes)
  - Defibrillation
  - Magnesium sulfate once stable
    - 2-4 gm SLOW IV at 1 g/min
  - Overdrive pacing
- Disopyramide toxicity
  - Although evidence is limited may consider Ca^{2+} administration
    - Adult: CaCl 10% 1 gm (10 mL) IV over 5-10 min; CaGluconate 10% 3 g (30 mL) IV over 5-10 min
    - Adult Infusion: 0.5 mEq/kg/hr = 0.2-0.4 mL/kg/hr of $CaCl_2$ (10%), or 0.6-1.2 mL/kg/hr of CaGluconate (10%)
    - Pediatric: CaCl 10% 10-20 mg/kg (0.1-0.2 mL/kg) IV over 10-15 min; CaGluconate 10% 20-50 mg/kg (0.2-0.5 mL/kg) IV over 5-10 min, not to exceed adult dose
    - Calcium chloride should only be administered via a Central line
- Propafenone toxicity
  - Isolated case reports suggest use of high-dose insulin for refractory poisoning but first-line therapy is sodium bicarbonate
  - Consider high-dose insulin/euglycemia therapy
    - Dextrose: ± 25-50 g (0.5-1 g/kg) IV bolus
    - Then: 0.25-0.5 g/kg/hr IV infusion
    - Insulin: 1 U/kg IV bolus regular human insulin
    - Then: 0.5-1.0 U/kg/hr IV infusion
      - Increase if no effect in 15 min
      - Titrate to 10 U/kg/hr
      - Monitor serum potassium because of intracellular shifts
      - Check capillary glucose q30min initially until stable, then check every 1-2 hrs

PEARL. Avoid Type IA, IC, and III antidysrhythmics

- Consider ILE or ECMO as salvage measures in CV collapse refractory to all other treatments

Disposition
- Observe minimum 6 hrs for regular release preparations
- Admit
  - Intentional ingestions of extended release preparations
  - Severe, persistent, or worsening signs and symptoms or those requiring antidotal treatment

Type III

Sources (used to prevent or terminate re-entrant dysrhythmias)
- Amiodarone
- Dronedarone
- Dofetilide
- Ibutilide
- Sotalol

Mechanism of Action
- Prolongation of cardiac myocyte repolarization by blockade of rapidly activating component of delayed rectifier K^+ channel
- Prolong both atrial and ventricular repolarization
- Amiodarone has weak α, β antagonism along with blocking Ca^{2+} channels and inactivated Na^+ channels

Clinical Manifestations
- Amiodarone
  - ACUTE
    - Prolongation of PR and QT intervals
      - Refractory VT or polymorphic VT
      - Sinus bradycardia
      - 1st degree AV block
  - CHRONIC
    - Interstitial pneumonitis: Most common extracardiac effect
    - Thyroid toxicity: Can cause hypothyroidism > thyrotoxicosis
    - Hepatic toxicity: Transaminitis and cirrhosis
    - Corneal toxicity—vision loss: Corneal deposits common
    - Gray or blue discoloration to sun-exposed skin
- Dofetilide/Ibutilide
  - QT prolongation
  - Development of ventricular dysrhythmias including polymorphic VT
  - Dofetilide: 3% incidence of torsades de pointes
  - Ibutilide: association with AKI

Treatment
- ABCDE
- Consider multi-dose activated charcoal
- Unstable VT/polymorphic VT
  — Cardioversion/defibrillation
  — Magnesium
    - 2-4 g SLOW IV at 1 g/min
  — Isoproterenol
    - Initiate @ 5 mcg/min; titrate by 1 mcg/min q5min to goal BP/HR
    - Usual dose 2-10 mcg/min
    - Duration ~ 10-15 min
  — Overdrive pacing should be initiated after defibrillation or spontaneous resolution of polymorphic VT

  > **PEARL.** Amiodarone-induced ventricular tachydysrhythmias, while uncommon, may be refractory to cardioversion and medications

- Correct electrolyte disturbances (potassium, calcium, magnesium)
- Consider ILE (amiodarone)
  — Loading dose 1.5 mL/kg 20% solution over 1 min
    - May repeat for persistent dysrhythmias
  — Infusion: 0.25 mL/kg/min for 3 min
- If beneficial response, continue infusion at 0.025 mL/kg/min
  — Infusion may be increased if BP declines
  — Max dose 10 mL/kg
- ECMO

Disposition
- Observe minimum 6 hrs
- Admit severe, persistent, or worsening signs and symptoms or those requiring antidotal treatment

ANTICOAGULANTS

Direct Oral Anticoagulants (DOACs)
Apixaban, Rivaroxaban, Edoxaban

Source
- Oral anticoagulant

Toxic Dose
- Risk exists with any ingestion

Mechanism of Action
- Selective direct Xa inhibitor

Clinical Manifestations
- Bleeding diathesis

Diagnostic
- PT/INR poor correlation with anticoagulant activity
- Anti Xa concentrations (availability depends on hospital lab)
- CBC

Treatment
- ABCDE
- Transfusion
- Activated charcoal
  - Generally not recommended because of risk of aspiration if patient deteriorates and literature does not clearly state an improved patient oriented outcome
- Prothrombin complex
  - Does not directly reverse Xa inhibitors
  - Potential risk of thromboembolism (controversial)
    - Difficult to determine if this is a true risk or just consequence of reversal in person with thrombotic disorder

  PEARL. Can fully reverse coagulopathy (normalize the INR) within 30 min and requires minimal volume as opposed to FFP

  - Activated PCC (FEIBA) or 4 factor PCC 25-50U/kg IV
- FFP
- Andexanet alfa
  - Recombinant, modified human factor Xa decoy protein (inactive Xa inhibitor) that binds to Xa inhibitors thereby inactivating them
  - Has been developed as antidote to reverse anticoagulation of oral direct and injected indirect factor "Xabans"

Disposition
Admit all with evidence of bleeding

Dabigatran

Source
- Oral anticoagulant

Toxic Dose
- Risk exists with any ingestion

Mechanism of Action
- Selective direct thrombin (IIa) inhibitor

Clinical Manifestations
- Bleeding diathesis

Diagnostics
- CBC
- BMP
- PT/INR poor correlation with anticoagulant activity
- Thrombin time (TT) may be useful
- Ecarin clotting time may be most precise but generally not available

Treatment
- ABCDE
- Transfusion
- Idarucizumab
    - Monoclonal antibody that binds dabigatran. Will bind both free and thrombin-bound dabigatran to neutralize its activity
    - Half-life ~45 min
    - In more than 90% of patients, inactivation of dabigatran lasted up to 12 hrs
    - Dosing
        - 2 separate vials (2.5 g each) given no greater than 15 min apart

    PEARL. Both vials should always be administered

    PEARL. Do not administer vitamin k if patient receiving idarucizumab

    PEARL. Rebound phenomenon seen in approximately 25% of study participants secondary to drug redistribution from tissues into the vascular compartment, resulting in re-elevation of TT/ECT (and relevant to our practice, re-elevation of TT and reappearance of clinically relevant bleeding)

- HD
    - 62-68% of drug can be removed in first 2-4 hrs
    - Effectiveness of HD to remove drug is controversial
    - Given the time required to initiate HD and if patient is hemodynamically unstable, this may not be a reasonable option

Disposition
Admit all with evidence of bleeding

Heparin (Unfractionated, LMWH) and Antiplatelets

Source
- Injectable anticoagulant medications

Toxic Dose
- Variable; risk of bleeding exists even with therapeutic doses

Mechanism of Action
- Heparin
  - Accelerates binding of antithrombin to thrombin and elevates PTT
  - Low molecular weight heparin: targeted activity against activated factor x with less against thrombin and so have minimal effect on PT
- Antiplatelet agents: Inhibit platelet IIb/IIIa and ADP receptors

Clinical Manifestations
- Heparin induced thrombocytopenia (HIT)
  - HIT 1 (also known as heparin associated thrombocytopenia [HAT])
    - Occurs within 48 hrs of initiation of heparin
    - Is not antibody induced
    - Recovers on its own in approximately 72 hrs
    - Patient can continue to receive heparin now or in the future
    - Post-operative thrombocytopenia falls under this category
  - HIT 2, HITT (heparin induced thrombocytopenia and thrombosis syndrome, a.k.a. white clot syndrome)
    - Antibody associated thrombocytopenia
    - Occurs multiple days (4-10) after administration of heparin

    PEARL. Unfractionated heparin has higher risk than LMWH

    - Platelet count falls by 50% or < 150
    - Associated with thrombotic events
    - Patient should not be given any form of heparin again
    - May be referred to as HITT if patient has thrombotic events

Pretest Scoring System for HIT: The 4 T's			
4 T's	2 points	1 point	0 points
Thrombocytopenia	Platelet count fall > 50% and platelet nadir ≥ 20	Platelet count fall 30-50% or platelet nadir 10-19	Platelet count fall < 30% or platelet nadir < 10
Timing of platelet count fall	Clear onset days 5-10 or platelet fall ≤1 day (prior heparin exposure within 30 days)	Consistent with days 5-10 fall, but unclear (missing platelet counts); onset after day 10; or fall ≤ 1 day (heparin exposure 30-100 days prior)	Platelet count fall < 4 days without recent exposure
Thrombosis/other sequelae	New thrombosis (confirmed); skin necrosis; acute systemic reaction post-IV UFH bolus	Progressive or recurrent thrombosis; non-necrotizing (erythematous) skin lesions; suspected thrombosis (unproven)	None
Other causes	None apparent	Possible	Definite

- Bleeding—most common
- Hyperkalemia
- Osteoporosis
- Elevated LFT

Diagnostics
- BMP
- LFT
- Bleeding
  - PTT for unfractionated heparin
  - Anti-factor Xa for LMWH and fondaparinux (requires specific calibration)

Treatment
- ABCDE
- HIT 1 or HAT
  - No treatment required
  - Platelet count will improve on its own
- HIT 2 or HITT
  - Stop heparin and switch to direct thrombin inhibitor or cautious use of fondaparinux

- Do not give prophylactic platelets if not actively bleeding for antiplatelet agents
  - Even if bleeding (intracranial hemorrhage), do not necessarily need to administer platelets
- Patient should not receive heparin again

PEARL. Do not administer low molecular weight heparin in the future if patient develops HIT2 or HITT after receiving unfractionated heparin

- Protamine
  - Used to reverse the effects of unfractionated and LMWH
  - 1 mg of protamine neutralizes approximately 100 units of UFH or 1mg of LMWH

Disposition
- Admit
  - Active or persistent bleeding
  - Development of HIT 2 or HITT

Warfarin

Source
- Anticoagulant medication

Toxic Dose
- Isolated dose of < 0.5 mg/kg in adults or children will not cause serious poisoning
  - In children
    - 0.5-0.7 mg/kg results in PT 1.5-2.5X normal
    - > 0.7 mg/kg results in excessive PT
- Delayed onset of action, effects may develop by 24 hrs, with full effect by 48-72 hrs

Mechanism of Action
- Inhibits vitamin K epoxide reductase, thereby blocking synthesis of clotting factors II, VII, IX, X, and regulatory proteins C, S

PEARL. Initiation of warfarin may produce a prothrombotic state because of relative protein C deficiency (concentrations fall first)

PEARL. Second generation hydroxycoumarin derivatives (brodifacoum) used as rat poisons. Depending on dose, can have prolonged effect (See Rodenticides chapter, p. 206)

- Patients who intentionally overdose on large amounts may be anticoagulated for months

PEARL. In April 2018, there were reported outbreaks of coagulopathy from synthetic cannabinoids adulterated with brodifacoum

Clinical Manifestations
- Bleeding
- Tissue necrosis
  - Very rare (< 0.1%)
  - Tends to occur in fatty tissues
  - Administer with heparin to avoid this
- Purple toe syndrome
  - Atherosclerotic plaques that embolize to distal microvasculature, causing ischemia after initiating warfarin
  - High risk of mortality

Diagnostics
- CBC
  - Intentional ingestions
- PT/PTT/INR

  PEARL. In pediatric exploratory ingestions if child is not bleeding, is well appearing, and presents shortly after ingestion, do not check coagulation studies. They will not be elevated and are unlikely to be clinically useful

- Reference labs can identify long-acting coumarins or superwarfarins
  - Tests take multiple days to return but may be useful for the patient with a coagulopathy of unknown etiology who denies ingesting these agents

Treatment
- ABCDE
- Life-threatening or severe bleeding
  - Prothrombin complex concentrate

    PEARL. More effective and preferred over FFP

    PEARL. Rapidly lowers INR in approximately 30 min

    - 25-50 U/kg IV depending on INR

- Elevated INR
  - Vitamin K1 (phytonadione)

  PEARL. **Administration may be either PO or IV, based on needed rate of reversal (subcutaneous route should be avoided)**
  - 5-10 mg PO or IV
  - IV dosing has more rapid onset of action but may cause anaphylactoid reaction
- FFP
  - Associated with standard risks of blood product transfusion
  - Volume required may prevent its use in patients with renal failure or congestive heart failure
  - Titrate to INR
  - May have to re-administer after 4-6 hrs
  - The lower the INR, the more FFP that needs to be administered to lower the INR further
  - The INR of FFP is approximately 1.4-1.6
- Intentional ingestions of long-acting hydroxycoumarins or superwarfarins
  - Adult intentional supratherapeutic ingestion: May require months of very high dose vitamin K

Disposition
- Admit
  - Active bleeding
  - Intentional ingestions
    - Can be followed by inpatient psychiatry if asymptomatic, serial INR measurements can be obtained and medical therapy provided (titration of vitamin K)

PEARL. **Single, accidental exposure to warfarin/superwarfarins in child does not result in toxicity; no treatment or follow-up is generally required**

CHEST Guidelines are included for chronic warfarin therapy with supratherapeutic INR. The chart below should not be utilized for warfarin overdose.

Condition	Description
INR above therapeutic range but < 5.0; no significant bleeding	Lower dose or omit dose, monitor more frequently, and resume at lower dose when INR therapeutic; if only minimally above therapeutic range, no dose reduction may be required (Grade 2C)
INR ≥ 5.0 but < 9.0; no significant bleeding	Omit next 1-2 doses, monitor more frequently, and resume at lower dose when INR in therapeutic range. Alternatively, omit dose and give vitamin K1 (< 5 mg orally), particularly if at increased risk of bleeding. If more rapid reversal is required because patient requires urgent surgery, vitamin K1 (2-4 mg orally) can be given with the expectation that a reduction of the INR will occur in 24 hrs. If INR still high, additional vitamin K1 (1-2 mg orally) can be given (Grade 2C)
	Hold warfarin therapy and give higher dose of vitamin K1 (5-10 mg orally) with the expectation that the INR will be reduced substantially in 24-48 hrs. Monitor more frequently and use additional vitamin K1 if INR > 9.0; no significant bleeding necessary. Resume therapy at lower dose when INR therapeutic (Grade 2C)
Serious bleeding at any elevation of INR	Hold warfarin therapy and give vitamin K1 (10 mg by slow IV infusion), supplemented with fresh plasma or prothrombin complex concentrate, depending on the urgency of the situation; recombinant factor VIIa may be considered as alternative to prothrombin complex concentrate; vitamin K1 can be repeated every 12 hrs (Grade 1)
Life-threatening bleeding	Hold warfarin therapy and give prothrombin complex concentrate supplemented with vitamin K1 (10 mg by slow IV infusion); recombinant factor VIIa may be considered as alternative to prothrombin complex concentrate; repeat if necessary, depending on INR (Grade 1C)

ANTICONVULSANTS

Note: Phenobarbital, See Sedative/Hypnotic chapter

Carbamazepine/Oxcarbazepine

Source
- Oral anti-epileptic medication

Toxic Dose
- Carbamazepine: > 10 mg/kg
- Oxcarbazepine
  - Adults: > 0.6-1.2 g
  - Children: > 8-10 mg/kg

Mechanism of Action
- Carbamazepine
  - Na^+ channel blockade
  - Anticholinergic
  - Adenosine antagonism
- Oxcarbazepine
  - Pro drug converted to carbamazepine analog

Clinical Manifestations
- ACUTE
  - CNS depression
  - Ataxia/nystagmus

    PEARL. Observed at serum carbamazepine concentration > 10 mg/L

  - Dystonia
  - N/V
  - Anticholinergic syndrome
  - QRS prolongation
  - QT prolongation
  - AV-blockade
  - Hypotension
  - Coma (waxing and waning mental status/cyclical coma)
  - Seizure (more likely with serum concentration > 40 mcg/mL)
- CHRONIC
  - Bone marrow suppression
  - Hyponatremia
  - Elevated LFT
  - Anticonvulsant hypersensitivity syndrome

Diagnostics
- Therapeutic concentrations
  - Carbamazepine 4-12 mg/L
  - Oxcarbazepine 1-3 mg/L
- Serial concentration every 2-3 hrs until peak
  - Carbamazepine erratic absorption
  - The active carbamazepine-10,11-epoxide metabolite is not detected in all assays that measure carbamazepine concentration
  - Oxcarbazepine does not cross-react with carbamazepine assay and concentration are not readily available

PEARL. Carbamazepine can produce false positive TCA on urine drug screen

Treatment
- ABCDE
- Seizures
  - Diazepam
    - Adult: 5-10 mg IV q5min PRN
    - Pediatric: 0.2 mg/kg IV q5min, max 10 mg
  - Lorazepam
    - Adult: 2-4 mg IV q15min PRN
    - Pediatric: 0.1 mg/kg IV, max 4 mg
      - Repeat 0.1 mg/kg q15min
  - Phenobarbital
    - 20 mg/kg IVPB
  - Propofol (if intubate)
    - 1-2 mg/kg IV bolus followed by continuous infusion 20 mcg/kg/min
- QRS prolongation and/or hypotension
  - Sodium bicarbonate
    - Bolus: 1-2 mEq/kg IVP over 1-2 min
    - Infusion: 100-150 mEq in 1 L D5W @ 150-200 mL/h (2x maintenance in pediatrics)
  - Lidocaine
    - Adult: 1-1.5 mg/kg IV x1 over 2 min; repeat 0.5 to 0.75 mg/kg bolus every 5-10 min (max cumulative dose: 3 mg/kg). Follow by infusion = 1-4 mg/min; titrate by 1-2 mg/min q10min
    - Pediatric: 1 mg/kg/dose; follow with continuous IV infusion 20-50 mcg/kg/minute. May administer second bolus if delay between initial bolus and start of infusion is > 15 min

Disposition
- Observe minimum 6 hrs
  - Controlled release preparations
- Admit
  - Intentional extended release ingestion
  - Severe, persistent, or worsening signs and symptoms or those requiring antidotal treatment

Gabapentin

Sources
- Oral anti-epileptic medication
- Sedative/hypnotic

Toxic Dose
- 91 g ingestion in an adult caused self-resolving dizziness, nystagmus, slurred speech

Mechanism of Action
- Derivative of GABA (designed to act as GABA agonist, but mechanism of action unknown)

Clinical Manifestations
- Sedation
- Ataxia
- Slurred speech
- Encephalopathy/ altered level of consciousness
- N/V

PEARL. Renal insufficiency/failure may result in increased toxicity or adverse effects from impaired elimination

Diagnostics
- No concentration clinically available

Treatment
- ABCDE
- Supportive care, airway protection
- With resolution of toxicity, monitor for acute withdrawal

Disposition
- Observe minimum 6 hrs
- Admit severe, persistent, or worsening signs and symptoms

Lacosamide

Source
- Oral and IV anti-epileptic medication

Toxic Dose
- No toxic dose established

Mechanism of Action
- Na^+ channel blockade

Clinical Manifestations
- ACUTE
  - CNS depression
  - Ataxia
  - QRS prolongation
  - QT prolongation
  - ST/T wave abnormalities
  - AV block
  - Hypotension

Diagnostics
- Therapeutic concentration 5-10 mg/L
- Limited data to suggest if serum concentrations are useful in guiding treatment or prognosis

Treatment
- ABCDE
- QRS prolongation and/or hypotension
  - Sodium bicarbonate
  - Bolus: 1-2 mEq/kg IVP over 1-2 min
  - Infusion: 100-150 mEq in 1 L D5W @ 150-200 mL/h (2x maintenance in pediatrics)
- Consider HD/CRRT

Disposition
- Observe minimum 6 hrs
- Admit severe, persistent, or worsening signs and symptoms or those requiring antidotal treatment

Lamotrigine

Source
- Oral anti-epileptic medication

Toxic Dose
- Concentrations > 14 mg/L
- Therapeutic range: 200-500 mg/day

Mechanism of Action
- Voltage-gated Na^+ channel blockade

Clinical Manifestations
- ACUTE
  - N/V
  - Ataxia
  - CNS depression
  - Nystagmus
  - Hypertonia
  - Seizures
  - Cardiac Na^+ channel blockade/QRS prolongation/ventricular dysrhythmias
- CHRONIC
  - Anticonvulsant hypersensitivity reaction
  - Rash with therapeutic use

Diagnostics
- Therapeutic concentration 3-14 mcg/mL
- Serum concentration may be available (likely institution dependent)
  - VPA increases adverse effects of lamotrigine and increases concentrations
- EKG

Treatment
- ABCDE
- Seizures
  - Diazepam
    - Adult: 5-10 mg IV q5min
    - Pediatric: 0.2 mg/kg IV q5min, max 10 mg
  - Lorazepam
    - Adult: 2-4 mg IV q15min PRN
    - Pediatric: 0.1 mg/kg IV, max 4 mg
      - Repeat 0.1 mg/kg in 10-15 min

- Phenobarbital
  - 15-20 mg/kg IVPB
- Propofol
  - 1 mg/kg IV, repeat 0.5 mg/kg IV PRN
- QRS prolongation and/or hypotension
  - IV sodium bicarbonate
    - Bolus: 1-2 mEq/kg IVP over 1-2 min
    - Infusion: 100-150 mEq in 1 L D5W @ 150-200 mL/h (2x maintenance in pediatrics)

Disposition
- Admit severe, persistent, or worsening signs and symptoms or those requiring antidotal treatment

Levetiracetam

Source
- Oral and IV anti-epileptic medication

Toxic Dose
- No toxic dose established

Mechanism of Action
- Pre-synaptic Ca^{2+} channel blockade

Clinical Manifestations
- ACUTE
  - CNS depression
  - Ataxia
  - Agitation/psychosis
  - Bradycardia
  - Hypotension
  - Leukopenia
  - Thrombocytopenia
- CHRONIC
  - Agitation (adolescents)

Diagnostics
- Therapeutic concentration 10-40 mg/L
- Serum concentration dependent on availability

Treatment
- ABCDE
- Consider HD/continuous renal replacement therapy for severe toxicity/coma
- Agitation/behavioral disturbance (adolescents)
  - Consider pyridoxine (vitamin B6): 50-100 mg PO daily

Disposition
- Observe minimum 6 hrs
- Admit severe, persistent, or worsening signs and symptoms

Phenytoin

Sources
- Oral or IV anti-epileptic medications

Toxic Dose
- Oral: 20 mg/kg
- IV: > 50 mg/min

Mechanism of Action
- Increases refractory period of voltage-gated Na^+ channels

Clinical Manifestations
- ACUTE (total)
  - > 20 mcg/mL: nystagmus
  - > 30 mcg/mL: slurred speech, ataxia, tremor
  - > 50 mcg/mL: confusion, coma

  PEARL. IV formulation of phenytoin (but not fosphenytoin) contains propylene glycol, which can cause cardiotoxicity with rapid infusion > 50 mg/min

- **Cardiac toxicity is not seen with oral overdose**
  - Hypotension
  - Bradycardia
  - Cardiac arrest
- CHRONIC
  - Hepatitis
  - Anticonvulsant hypersensitivity reaction

  PEARL. Gingival hyperplasia (Rx: folic acid)

  - Teratogenic

Diagnostics
- Therapeutic concentration 10-20 mg/L
- Serial phenytoin concentration until down trending; correct based on albumin
  — Corrected phenytoin = total phenytoin/[(0.2 × albumin) + 0.1]

PEARL. Free phenytoin concentration if clinical toxicity suspected in low protein states

Treatment
- ABCDE
- Supportive care; fall prevention

Disposition
- Observe minimum 6 hrs
- Admit severe, persistent, or worsening signs and symptoms

Pregabalin

Source
- Oral anti-epileptic medication

Toxic Dose
- No known toxic dose
- Reports of dosages as high as 8000 mg in clinical development trials without notable clinical consequences

Mechanism of Action
- More potent analog of gabapentin

Clinical Manifestations
- Therapeutic concentration 2.8-8.3 mg/L
- ACUTE
  — Drowsiness
  — Dizziness
  — Tremor
  — Potential drug of abuse
- CHRONIC
  — Peripheral edema
  — Weight gain
  — Decompensated CHF

Treatment
- ABCDE

Disposition
- Observe minimum 6 hrs
- Admit severe, persistent, or worsening signs and symptoms

Tiagabine

Source
- Oral anti-epileptic medication

Toxic Dose
- Limited data; trials have shown toxicity at doses > 400 mg

Mechanism of Action
- Inhibits reuptake of GABA

Clinical Manifestations
- Therapeutic concentrations 0.01-0.1 mg/L
- ACUTE
  - Facial myoclonus
  - Nystagmus
  - Lethargy
  - Seizures, status epilepticus (both in therapeutic dosing and overdose)

Treatment
- ABCDE
- Seizures
  - Diazepam
    - Adult: 5-10 mg IV q5-10min PRN
    - Pediatric: 0.2-0.5 mg/kg IV q5-10min
  - Lorazepam
    - Adult: 2-4 mg IV q10-15min PRN
    - Pediatric: 0.05-0.1 mg/kg IV q10-15min PRN
  - Phenobarbital
    - 130-260 mg IV q20min titrate to effect (in adults)
    - 10 mg/kg IVPB may require secure airway
  - Propofol (if intubated)
    - Continuous infusion of 5 mcg/kg/min titrate (rec. max of 55 mcg/kg/min)

Disposition
- Observe minimum 6 hrs
- Admit severe, persistent, or worsening signs and symptoms

Topiramate

Source
- Oral anti-epileptic medication

Toxic Dose
- Unclear, but higher incidence of adverse effects seen at > 400 mg/day

Mechanism of Action
- Voltage-gated Na^+ channel blockade
- Carbonic anhydrase inhibitor, enhances GABA
- Decreases activation of glutamate receptors

Clinical Manifestations
- ACUTE
  - Somnolence, coma, seizures

  PEARL. Hyperchloremic non-anion gap metabolic acidosis
- CHRONIC
  - Renal stones (calcium phosphate)
  - Glaucoma

Diagnostics
- Serum concentration
  - Therapeutic concentration 5-25 mg/L
- BMP

  PEARL. Can increase the effects of valproic acid

Treatment
- ABCDE
- Correct electrolyte abnormalities
- Ensure resolution of metabolic acidosis
- IV sodium bicarbonate for QRS prolongation and/or hypotension

Disposition
- Observe minimum 6 hrs
- Admit severe, persistent, or worsening signs and symptoms

Valproic Acid

Source
- Oral or IV anti-epileptic medications

Toxic Dose
- ACUTE ingestion
  - > 200 mg/kg

PEARL. CHRONIC toxicity possible with therapeutic concentration

Mechanism of Action
- Increases GABA
- Prolongs recovery of inactivated Na^+ channels

PEARL. Impairs beta-oxidation and disrupts urea cycle

Clinical Manifestations
- ACUTE
  - N/V
  - CNS depression
  - AG metabolic acidosis
  - Hypotension
  - Pancreatitis

  PEARL. Hyperammonemia

- CHRONIC
  - Microvesicular steatosis
  - Pancreatitis
  - Hypocalcemia
  - Hypernatremia
  - Pancytopenia
  - Hyperammonemia

Diagnostics
- Therapeutic concentration 50-150 mg/L

PEARL. Delayed absorption with extended release formulations and in overdose

  - Serial valproic acid concentrations until falling
  - NH_3
  - LFT
  - BMP
  - CBC
  - Ca^{2+}

Treatment

> **PEARL.** L-carnitine for encephalopathy + hyperammonemia

- Consider 100 mg/kg IV (max 6 g) over 15-30 min, then 15 mg/kg (max 3 g per dose) IV q4hrs over 10-30 min
- Serum concentration > 850 mg/L, coma, hemodynamic instability
  - Hemodialysis may be useful due to increased free/unbound drug

Disposition
- Observe minimum 6 hrs
- Admit severe, persistent, or worsening signs and symptoms or those requiring antidotal treatment

Vigabatrin

Source
- Oral anti-epileptic medication

Toxic Dose
- No toxic dose established

Mechanism of Action
- Irreversible inhibitor of GABA-transaminase

Clinical Manifestations
- Agitation
- Psychosis
- Sedation
- Coma

Diagnostics
- Therapeutic concentration 20-80 mg/L
- Serum concentration not readily available

Treatment
- ABCDE

Disposition
- Observe minimum 6 hrs
- Admit severe, persistent, or worsening signs and symptoms

Zonisamide

Source
- Oral anti-epileptic medication

Toxic Dose
- No toxic dose established

Mechanism of Action
- Inhibits carbonic anhydrase

Clinical Manifestations
- Hypotension
- Somnolence
- Coma

Diagnostics
- Therapeutic concentration 10-40 mg/L

Treatment
- ABCDE

Disposition
- Observe minimum 6 hrs
- Admit severe, persistent, or worsening signs and symptoms

ANTIDEPRESSANTS

Lithium

Source
- Oral medication for psychiatric disorders
- OTC herbal products

Toxic Dose
- Toxic effects as low as 1.5 mEq/L

> **PEARL.** Lithium is rapidly absorbed and slowly redistributed, thus concentration measured shortly after ingestion can be elevated, but may drop after equilibrium reached. Obtain lithium concentration at 6 hrs after ingestion for more accurate measurement, and follow serial concentration until peak.

Mechanism of Action
- Cation that enters cells and substitutes for Na⁺ or K⁺
- Alters serotonin and norepinephrine uptake via complex mechanism involving alteration in cell signaling

Clinical Manifestations
- GI (occur in acute and acute-on-chronic toxicity)
  - N/V/D
- CNS (occur in chronic, acute-on-chronic and late acute toxicity)
  - Ataxia
  - Nystagmus
  - Clonus
  - Hyperreflexia
  - Tremor
  - Seizures
  - Coma
  - Serotonin syndrome (See p. 247)
  - SILENT (Syndrome of irreversible lithium-effectuated neurotoxicity) irreversible neurologic and neuropsychiatric abnormalities
- CV
  - Bradycardia
  - Non-specific T-wave changes (flattening and inversion in precordial leads)
  - Significant hemodynamic compromise is unlikely
- Endocrine/Metabolic
  - Hypothyroidism
  - Hyperthyroidism
  - Hyperparathyroidism
  - Nephrogenic diabetes insipidus

PEARL. Hypothyroidism is the most common endocrine abnormality caused by lithium

Diagnostics
- Serum lithium concentrations (falsely elevated concentration may occur if using green-top lithium-containing tubes)
  - Therapeutic range = 0.6-1.2 mEq/L
  - Serial concentration
  - Must be correlated clinically

PEARL. Resolution of clinical signs of toxicity may lag behind falls in serum lithium oncentration

- EKG
- CBC

    PEARL. Leukocytosis associated with lithium use

- BMP
- TSH

Treatment
- ABCDE
- IVF NSS at 2X-maintenance
  - Ensure serum sodium is normal
  - Volume resuscitation
- Stop medications that impair renal function or contribute to hyponatremia
  - ACE
  - Diuretics
- Consider whole bowel irrigation in acute massive ingestion
- HD
  - Presence of decreased level of consciousness, seizures or dysrhythmias irrespective of lithium concentration
  - Significant signs of toxicity with acute renal failure impairing effective elimination
  - Extracorporeal Treatments in Poisoning Workgroup recommends HD for lithium concentration > 4 mEq/L and elevated creatinine or lithium > 5 mEq/L
    - This recommendation is based on limited low-level evidence
    - Decision to dialyze should be made based on clinical signs of toxicity

Disposition
- Observe minimum 6 hrs
- Admit severe, persistent, or worsening signs and symptoms or rising concentrations or requiring HD

Monoamine Oxidase Inhibitors (MAOIs)

Toxic Dose
- 2-3 mg/kg of first-generation MAOI
  - Potentially life-threatening

    PEARL. Because MAOIs are irreversible, adverse drug interactions may occur up to 2 weeks after discontinuation, if pro-serotonergic agents are started

Mechanism of Action
- MAO inhibitors inactivate MAO (monoamine oxidase), an enzyme responsible for degradation of catecholamines within CNS neurons
- Leads to increased catecholamines and hyperadrenergic manifestations
- MAOIs are rarely used except in cases of refractory depression or Parkinson's
- Irreversible non-selective MAOIs are famous for extensive drug and food interactions (tyramine reaction)

First Generation—Irreversible & Nonselective
  - Tranylcypromine, isocarboxazid, or phenelzine

Second Generation—Irreversible & Selective
  - Chlorgyline, selegiline

Third Generation—Selective & Reversible
  - Moclobemide (unavailable in the U.S.)

Other Drugs with MOA properties
  - Procarbazine, linezolid, MDMA, methylene blue, St. John's Wort (*Hypericum perforatum*)

Clinical Manifestations
- **Acute overdose**

  PEARL. Onset of toxicity can be delayed

  PEARL. Biphasic response. Initial CNS excitation & peripheral sympathetic stimulation that leads to coma and rapid CV collapse

- Food (tyramine) interactions and drug/drug interactions (SSRIs)
  - Occurs within minutes to hours
  - Headache, tachycardia, hypertension, ischemia, altered mental status
  - Serotonin syndrome (See Serotonin Syndrome, p. 247)
  - Sympathomimetic toxidrome (See Sympathomimetics, p. 238)

Diagnostics

PEARL. Selegiline is metabolized to L-methamphetamine and L-amphetamine and may be detectable on urine drug screens

Treatment
- ABCDE
- Acute overdose
  - Hyperthermia
    - Rapid cooling (normal core temp in < 30 min)
    - Requires control of motor hyperactivity and prevention of shivering

- Agitation/Seizures
  - Diazepam
    - Adult: 5-10 mg IV q5-10min PRN
    - Pediatric: 0.2-0.5 mg/kg IV q5-10min
  - Lorazepam
    - Adult: 2-4 mg IV q10-15min PRN
    - Pediatric: 0.05-0.1 mg/kg IV q10-15min PRN
  - Phenobarbital
    - 130-260 mg IV q20min titrate to effect (in adults)
    - 10 mg/kg IVPB may require secure airway
  - Propofol (if intubated)
    - Continuous infusion of 5 mcg/kg/min titrate (rec. max of 55 mcg/kg/min)
- Hypertension
  - Nitroprusside, nitroglycerin, phentolamine
  - β-adrenergic antagonists are contra-indicated
- Hypotension
  - IVF
  - Vasopressors
    - Epinephrine
      - Infusion: Initial 0.05-2 mcg/kg/min Titrate by 0.02-0.05 mcg/kg/min q15min to goal MAP
      - No true max; higher dosing may be required
    - Norepinephrine
      - Infusion: 0.05 mcg/kg/min, then titrate by 0.02 mcg/kg/min q5min to goal MAP
      - No true max and higher dosing may be required
    - Vasopressin
      - 0.01 U/min titrate to goal MAP
    - Phenylephrine
      - Initiate 100-180 mcg /min, then titrate to goal MAP

- **Drug/drug interactions or food interactions**
  - Discontinue medications/foods
  - Serotonin syndrome (See Serotonin Syndrome, p. 247)
  - Sympathomimetic toxidrome (See Sympathomimetics, p. 238)
- **Withdrawal**
  - Can begin 24-72 hrs after stopping use
  - Symptoms include GI distress, agitation, psychosis, seizures
  - Treatment is supportive care and possibly benzodiazepines
  - Consider restarting medication if indicated

Disposition
- Admit severe, persistent, or worsening signs and symptoms

  PEARL. Because of potential for delayed onset of toxicity, admit all intentional exposures to ICU even if asymptomatic

Selective Serotonin Reuptake Inhibitors (SSRIs), Selective Norepinephrine Reuptake Inhibitors (SNRIs), Norepinephrine Dopamine Reuptake Inhibitors (NDRIs)

Source
- Antidepressant medication

Toxic Dose
- Generally well-tolerated, even in larger overdoses

Mechanism of Action
- SSRIs: Selectively inhibit serotonin reuptake
- SNRIs: Selectively inhibit serotonin and norepinephrine reuptake
- NDRIs: Inhibit reuptake of norepinephrine and dopamine
  - Peripheral α-adrenergic blockade: trazodone, mirtazapine

Clinical Manifestations
- GI
  - N/V
- CNS
  - Ataxia
  - Sedation
  - Seizure
    - Citalopram, escitalopram—often within first few hours
    - Venlafaxine, desvenlafaxine
  - Coma
  - Serotonin syndrome (See Serotonin Syndrome, p. 247)
- CV
  - Dizzy/lightheaded
  - Hypotension: trazodone
  - Sinus tachycardia
  - QRS prolongation: venlafaxine
  - QT prolongation resulting in torsades de pointes—can be delayed
    - Citalopram (escitalopram is less cardiotoxic)

Diagnostics
- EKG

Treatment
- ABCDE
- Seizure
  - Diazepam
    - Adult: 5-10 mg IV q5-10min PRN
    - Pediatric: 0.2-0.5 mg/kg IV q5-10min
  - Lorazepam
    - Adult: 2-4 mg IV q10-15min PRN
    - Pediatric: 0.05-0.1 mg/kg IV q10-15min PRN
  - Phenobarbital
    - 130-260 mg IV q20min titrate to effect (in adults)
    - 10 mg/kg IVPB may require secure airway
  - Propofol (if intubated)
    - Continuous infusion of 5 mcg/kg/min titrate (rec. max of 55 mcg/kg/min)
- QRS prolongation
  - Sodium bicarbonate
    - Bolus: 1-2 mEq/kg IVP over 1-2 min
    - Infusion: 100-150 mEq in 1 L D5W @ 150-200 mL/hr (2x maintenance in pediatrics)
- Torsades de pointes
  - Magnesium
    - 2-4 gm IV slow 1 mg/min
- Overdrive pacing
  - Serotonin Syndrome (See Serotonin Syndrome, p. 247)

Disposition
- Observe minimum 6 hrs
- Admit
  - Severe, persistent, or worsening signs and symptoms or those requiring antidotal treatment
  - All sustained release venlafaxine and bupropion
  - Citalopram > 600 mg and escitalopram > 300 mg ingestion
    - Prolonged observation may be warranted because of reports of delayed onset cardiotoxicity

Tricyclic Antidepressants (TCAs)

Source
- Antidepressant medication

Toxic Dose
- 10-20 mg/kg (therapeutic dose 2-4 mg/kg/day)
- Adults: Ingestion > 1 g usually associated with life-threatening effects
- Children: 5 mg/kg may present with clinical toxicity

Mechanism of Action
- Inhibit presynaptic reuptake of norepinephrine and/or serotonin
- Inhibit cardiac Na$^+$ channels "membrane stabilizing effect"
- Competitive inhibition of muscarinic acetylcholine receptors
- Peripheral α-adrenergic blockade
- GABA$_A$ antagonism
- K$^+$ channel blockade inhibiting K$^+$ efflux

Clinical Manifestations
- Significant signs of toxicity typically develop within 6 hrs of ingestion
- Anticholinergic toxidrome (See Toxidrome Table, p. 282)
- CV

    PEARL. Sinus tachycardia most common finding

    — EKG can demonstrate:
    - Rightward axis
    - Right bundle branch block pattern
    - QRS prolongation
    - QT prolongation
    - Terminal R-wave (> 3 mm) in aVR
    - Terminal R-wave/S-wave ratio of > 0.7 mm in aVR
    - Brugada pattern (rare finding)
    - Myocardial depression and vasodilation leads to refractory hypotension—most common cause of death
    - Ventricular arrhythmias

    — Hypotension

    PEARL. Precipitous fall in pH may result in worsening cardiotoxicity

- CNS
    — Delirium—secondary to anti-muscarinic effects
    — Mental status depression and coma
    — Seizures

PEARL. Seizures are usually generalized and brief, most often occur within 1-2 hrs of ingestion

Diagnostics
- EKG
- CXR
- BMP
- VBG/ABG

Treatment
- ABCDE

PEARL. Do not use flumazenil or physostigmine

- QRS prolongation
  - Sodium bicarbonate
    - Bolus: 1-2 mEq/kg IV push over 1-2 min—repeat as necessary every 3-5 min to narrow the QRS interval
    - May require large amounts of sodium bicarbonate
    - Bolus doses are preferred over sodium bicarbonate infusion
    - Infusion: 100-150 mEq in 1 L D5W @ 150-200 mL/h (2x maintenance in pediatrics)

    PEARL. Target serum < pH 7.55, [Na$^+$] 150 mEq/L

  - Lidocaine—can be considered for dysrhythmias or persistent cardiotoxicity despite sodium bicarbonate treatment
    - Adult: 1-1.5 mg/kg IV push × 1 over 2 min; follow by infusion at 1-4 mg/min; titrate by 1-2 mg/min q10min. Infusion rate 20-50 mcg/kg/min
    - Pediatric: 1 mg/kg; follow with infusion at 20-50 mcg/kg/min. May administer second bolus if delay between initial bolus and start of infusion is > 15 min
    - Do not exceed 20 mcg/kg/min in patients with shock, hepatic disease, cardiac arrest or CHF

    PEARL. Avoid Class IA (quinidine, procainamide, disopyramide) and Class IC antiarrhythmics (flecainide, propafenone)—may worsen Na$^+$ channel inhibition

    - **Avoid use of Class III (amiodarone, sotalol) antiarrhythmics**
- Torsades de pointes
  - Uncommon in acute toxicity
  - Treatment: 2-4 g magnesium sulfate IV slow at 1 mg/min
  - Overdrive pacing

- Seizures
  - Diazepam
    - Adult: 5-10 mg IV q5-10min PRN
    - Pediatric: 0.2-0.5 mg/kg IV q5-10min
  - Lorazepam
    - Adult: 2-4 mg IV q10-15min PRN
    - Pediatric: 0.05-0.1 mg/kg IV q10-15min
  - Phenobarbital
    - 130-260 mg IV q20min titrate to effect (in adults)
    - 10 mg/kg IVPB may require secure airway
  - Propofol (if intubated)
    - Continuous infusion of 5 mcg/kg/min titrate (rec. max of 55 mcg/kg/min)
- Refractory toxicity/shock
  - Vasopressors
    - Epinephrine
      - Infusion: Initial 0.05-2 mcg/kg/min. Titrate by 0.02-0.05 mcg/kg/min q15min to goal MAP
      - No true max and higher dosing may be required
    - Norepinephrine
      - Infusion: 0.05 mcg/kg/min, then titrate by 0.02 mcg/kg/min q5min to goal MAP
      - No true max and higher dosing may be required
  - ILE
    - If above methods fail/refractory shock
    - Loading dose 1.5 mL/kg 20% solution over 1 min
      - May repeat for persistent dysrhythmias
    - Infusion: 0.25 mL/kg/min over 30-60 min
  - ECMO
    - If prior methods fail/refractory shock

Disposition

- Observe minimum 6 hrs
- Admit severe, persistent, or worsening signs and symptoms or those requiring antidotal treatment

Atypical Antidepressants: Bupropion

Sources
- Antidepressant medications
- Smoking cessation aids

Toxic Dose
- Doses > 450 mg/day may increase risk of seizures

Mechanism of Action
- Inhibition of the reuptake of dopamine and norepinephrine

Clinical Manifestations
- GI
  — N/V
- CNS
  — Tremors
  — Agitation
  — Seizures

  PEARL. Seizures can occur at therapeutic dosing or overdose and may be delayed with extended release preparations (up to 24 hrs)

- CV
  — Sinus tachycardia
  — HTN
  — QRS prolongation (thought to be from gap junction inhibition not Na^+ channel inhibition)

Diagnostics
- EKG

Treatment
- ABCDE
- Seizures/agitation
  — Diazepam
    - Adult: 5-10 mg IV q5-10min PRN
    - Pediatric: 0.2-0.5 mg/kg IV q5-10min
  — Lorazepam
    - Adult: 2-4 mg IV q10-15min PRN
    - Pediatric: 0.05-0.1 mg/kg IV q10-15min PRN

- Phenobarbital
  - 130-260 mg IV q20min titrate to effect (in adults)
  - 10 mg/kg IVPB may require secure airway
- Propofol (if intubated)
  - Continuous infusion of 5 mcg/kg/min titrate (rec. max of 55 mcg/kg/min)
- QRS prolongation
  - Sodium bicarbonate can be tried but may not be effective
    - Bolus: 1-2 mEq/kg IVP over 1-2 min
    - Infusion: 100-150 mEq in 1 L D5W @ 150-200 mL/h (2x maintenance in pediatrics)
    - Target serum pH 7.45-7.55
- ILE
  - Loading dose 1.5 mL/kg 20% solution over 2-3 min
    - May be repeated twice at q5min intervals for persistent cardiac instability
    - Max dose of 12mL/kg in 60 min
  - Infusion: 0.25-0.5 mL/kg/min over 30-60 min
- ECMO
  - For refractory cardiogenic shock/arrest

Disposition

- Observe minimum 6 hrs for immediate release formulations
- Admit
  - Severe, persistent, or worsening signs and symptoms or those requiring antidotal treatment
  - All intentional ingestions of sustained or extended release formulations

ANTIDIABETICS AND HYPOGLYCEMICS

α-Glucosidase Inhibitors

Sources
- Drugs used to treat diabetes (acarbose, miglitol, etc.)

Toxic Dose
- Low toxicity

Mechanism of Action
- Inhibits α-glucosidase enzymes in the small intestine, preventing cleavage of disaccharides (sucrose) and oligosaccharides

Clinical Manifestations
- Hypoglycemia unlikely
- GI symptoms
  - N/V/D
  - Bloating
  - Flatulence
  - Abdominal pain
  - Elevated LFTs with acarbose

Diagnostics
- Blood glucose q2hrs

Treatment
- Food/drink PO ad lib
- IV or oral dextrose if hypoglycemic
  - Oral glucose gel or tablets available while securing IV access
  - D5W or D10W infusion titrated to maintain euglycemia
    - 0.5-1.0 g/kg, adjust based on size
  - If concentration > D12.5W central venous access needed
    - Adult: D50 (0.5 g/mL) IV
    - Pediatric: D25 (0.25 g/mL) IV
    - Neonates: D10 (0.1 g/mL) IV
  - Goal to maintain glucose in normal range (70-110 mg/dL)

Disposition
- Observe minimum 6 hrs
- Admit severe, persistent, or worsening signs and symptoms or those requiring antidotal treatment

Amylin Analog

Sources
- Drugs used to treat diabetes (pramlintide)

Toxic Dose
- Hypoglycemia not expected from drug alone; possible when given with another hypoglycemic agent

Mechanism of Action
- Inhibits endogenous glucagon secretion and slows gastrointestinal motility to prolong satiety
- Duration of action: 3 hrs

Clinical Manifestations
- Hypoglycemia unlikely

Diagnostics
- Blood glucose q2hrs

Treatment
- Food/drink PO ad lib
- IV or oral dextrose if hypoglycemic
  - Oral glucose gel or tablets available while securing IV access
  - D5W or D10W infusion titrated to maintain euglycemia
    - 0.5-1.0 g/kg, adjust based on size
  - If concentration > D12.5W central venous access needed
    - Adult: D50 (0.5 g/mL) IV
    - Pediatric: D25 (0.25 g/mL) IV
    - Neonates: D10 (0.1 g/mL) IV
  - Goal to maintain glucose in normal range (70-110 mg/dL)

Disposition
- Observe minimum 6 hrs
- Admit severe, persistent, or worsening signs and symptoms or those requiring antidotal treatment

Biguanides

Sources
- Drugs used to treat diabetes (metformin, phenformin)

Toxic Dose
- Metformin: Lactemia occurred 9 hrs after 25 g ingestion in 83-year-old; cardiac arrest and lactemia occurred 4 hrs after 35 g ingestion in 33-year-old

Mechanism of Action
- Inhibits gluconeogenesis
- Stimulates peripheral glucose uptake
- Inhibits complex I in the mitochondrial electron transport chain

Clinical Manifestations
- GI
  - N/V/D
  - Abdominal pain
- Metabolic
  - Anion gap metabolic acidosis
  - Lactemia

PEARL. Metformin-associated metabolic acidosis (MALA) with lactemia in those with large overdose, renal, or hepatic disease

- Hypoglycemia rarely reported as no stimulation of endogenous insulin release

Diagnostics
- Blood glucose q2hrs
- BMP
- Lactate, repeat q6hrs to trend

Treatment
- Supportive and symptomatic care, IVFs, anti-emetics
- MALA
  - Thiamine IV
  - IV sodium bicarbonate
    - Bolus: 1-2 mEq/kg IVP over 1-2 min
    - Infusion: 100-150 mEq in 1 L D5W @ 150-200 mL/h (2x maintenance in pediatrics)
  - Hemodialysis
    - Severe or refractory acidosis
    - Renal failure
    - Clinical decompensation despite supportive care

Disposition
- Observe minimum 6 hrs
- Admit severe, persistent or worsening signs and symptoms or those requiring antidotal treatment

DPP-4 Inhibitors

Sources
- Drugs used to treat diabetes (alogliptin, linagliptin, saxagliptin, sitagliptin)

Toxic Dose
- Sitagliptin: 700 mg ingestion caused abdominal pain but no hypoglycemia
- Sitagliptin: 1800 mg ingestion caused no symptoms in 70-year-old woman

Mechanism of Action
- Inhibit metabolism of endogenous GLP-1 (no effect on pharmaceutical GLP-1 agonists)
- Duration of action: 24 hrs

Clinical Manifestations
- Hypoglycemia unlikely but sparse data in overdose setting
- Angioedema (DPP-4 is involved in bradykinin metabolism)

Diagnostics
- Blood glucose q2hrs

Treatment
- Food/drink PO ad lib
- IV or oral dextrose if hypoglycemic
  - Oral glucose gel or tablets available while securing IV access
  - D5W or D10W infusion titrated to maintain euglycemia
    - 0.5-1.0 g/kg, adjust based on size
  - If concentration > D12.5W central venous access needed
    - Adult: D50 (0.5 g/mL) IV
    - Pediatric: D25 (0.25 g/mL) IV
    - Neonates: D10 (0.1 g/mL) IV
  - Goal to maintain glucose in normal range (70-110 mg/dL)

Disposition
- Observe minimum 6 hrs
- Admit severe, persistent, or worsening signs and symptoms or those requiring antidotal treatment

GLP-1 Analogs

Sources
- Drugs used to treat diabetes (albiglutide, dulaglutide, exenatide, liraglutide, lixisenatide, teduglutide)

Toxic Dose
- Exenatide: 1800 mcg injection caused nausea
- Liraglutide: 17.4 mg caused nausea/vomiting; no hypoglycemia reported

Mechanism of Action
- Stimulate insulin secretion in glucose-dependent fashion
- Inhibits glucagon secretion
- Slows gastric emptying
- Increases satiety
- Duration of action: variable based on agent and route, hours to days

Clinical Manifestations
- Hypoglycemia unlikely but sparse data in overdose setting

Diagnostics
- Blood glucose q2hrs

Treatment
- Food/drink PO ad lib
- IV or oral dextrose if hypoglycemic
  - Oral glucose gel or tablets available while securing IV access
  - D5W or D10W infusion titrated to maintain euglycemia
    - 0.5-1.0 g/kg, adjust based on size
  - If concentration > D12.5W central venous access needed
    - Adult: D50 (0.5 g/mL) IV
    - Pediatric: D25 (0.25 g/mL) IV
    - Neonates: D10 (0.1 g/mL) IV
  - Goal to maintain glucose in normal range (70-110 mg/dL)

Disposition
- Observe minimum 6 hrs
- Admit severe, persistent, or worsening signs and symptoms or those requiring antidotal treatment

Insulin

Sources
- Rapid acting (aspart, glulisine, lispro)—onset 15-30 min, duration 3-5 hrs
- Short acting (Regular)—onset 30-60 min, duration 4-8 hrs
- Intermediate acting (NPH)—onset 1-3 hrs, duration 18-24 hrs
- Long acting (degludec, detemir, glargine)—onset 1-3 hrs, duration 24+ hrs

Toxic Dose
- Narrow therapeutic index and depends on multiple clinical factors
- 800-3200 units: Profound hypoglycemia and neurologic injury has occurred

Mechanism of Action
- Exogenous insulin stimulates peripheral glucose uptake
- Inhibits gluconeogenesis

Clinical Manifestations
- CNS
  - Confusion
- Metabolic
  - Hypoglycemia
  - Hypokalemia
  - Hypophosphatemia

Diagnostics
- Blood glucose q2hrs while awake, q1hr when asleep
- BMP
- Phosphate

Treatment
- Food/drink PO ad lib
- IV or oral dextrose if hypoglycemic
  - Oral glucose gel or tablets available while securing IV access
  - D5W or D10W infusion titrated to maintain euglycemia
    - 0.5-1.0 g/kg, adjust based on size
  - If concentration > D12.5W central venous access needed
    - Adult: D50 (0.5 g/mL) IV
    - Pediatric: D25 (0.25 g/mL) IV
    - Neonates: D10 (0.1 g/mL) IV
  - Goal to maintain glucose in normal range (70-110 mg/dL)
    - In non-type 1 diabetics over-treatment resulting in hyperglycemia may result in hyperinsulinemia and possible rebound hypoglycemia
- Correct hypokalemia, hypomagnesemia, hypocalcemia
- Replete thiamine if deficient
- Octreotide
  - 1-2 mcg/kg SC, max 50 mcg q6hrs
  - Although data limited, may be of benefit in non-Type-1 diabetics with refractory hypoglycemia

Disposition
- Admit
  - All intentional insulin overdoses because of risk of depot effect and delayed/recurrent hypoglycemia
  - All long acting insulin overdoses
  - Severe, persistent, or worsening signs and symptoms or those requiring antidotal treatment
- Feed and observe 4-6 hrs unintentional rapid/short/intermediate insulin injections
- Observe 6 hrs unintentional rapid/short/intermediate insulin injections and feed ad lib
- Discharge asymptomatic and euglycemic

Meglitinides

Sources
- Drugs used to treat diabetes (nateglinide, repaglinide)

Toxic Dose
- Repaglinide: 4 mg ingestion caused hypoglycemia in non-diabetic 18-year-old
- Nateglinide: 3420 mg ingestion caused hypoglycemia for 6 hrs in non-diabetic adult

Mechanism of Action
- Same as sulfonylureas

Clinical Manifestations
- Similar to insulin
- Because of shorter duration of action compared to sulfonylurea, may not cause protracted hypoglycemia

Diagnostics
- Blood glucose q2hrs while awake, q1hr when asleep
- BMP

Treatment
- Food/drink PO ad lib
- IV or oral dextrose if hypoglycemic
  - Oral glucose as gel or tablets available while establishing IV access
  - D5W or D10W infusion titrated to maintain euglycemia
    - 0.5-1.0 g/kg, adjust based on size

- If concentration > D12.5W central venous access needed
  - Adult: D50 (0.5 g/mL) IV
  - Pediatric: D25 (0.25 g/mL) IV
  - Neonates: D10 (0.1 g/mL) IV
- Goal is to maintain glucose in normal range (70-110 mg/dL)
- Octreotide
  - 1-2 mcg/kg SC, max 50 mcg q6hrs
- Correct hypokalemia, hypomagnesemia, hypocalcemia
- Replete thiamine if deficient

Disposition
- Observe minimum 6 hrs
- Admit severe, persistent, or worsening signs and symptoms or those requiring antidotal treatment

SGLT-2 Inhibitors

Sources
- Drugs used to treat diabetes (canagliflozin, dapagliflozin, empagliflozin)

Toxic Dose
- Toxic dose undetermined

Mechanism of Action
- Prevent glucose reuptake in the kidneys
- Duration of action: unavailable, but half-life 10-13 hrs

Clinical Manifestations
- Hypoglycemia unlikely but sparse data in overdose setting
- Hypovolemia because of osmotic diuresis

PEARL. Euglycemic diabetic ketoacidosis reported

Diagnostics
- Blood glucose q2hrs
- BMP
- Serum acetone, beta-hydroxybutyrate
- UA

Treatment
- IVF
- IV insulin (euglycemic DKA)

- IV dextrose if hypoglycemic
  - Oral glucose gel or tablets available while securing IV access
  - D5W or D10W infusion titrated to maintain euglycemia
    - 0.5-1.0 g/kg, adjust based on size
  - If concentration > D12.5W central venous access needed
    - Adult: D50 (0.5 g/mL) IV
    - Pediatric: D25 (0.25 g/mL) IV
    - Neonates: D10 (0.1 g/mL) IV
  - Goal to maintain glucose in normal range (70-110 mg/dL)

Disposition
- Observe minimum 6 hrs
- Admit
  - DKA
  - Severe, persistent, or worsening signs and symptoms or those requiring antidotal treatment

Sulfonylureas

Sources
- Drugs used to treat diabetes (chlorpropamide, glimepiride, glipizide, glyburide, tolbutamide)

Toxic Dose
- Chlorpropamide: 250 mg
- Glipizide: 5 mg
- Glyburide
  - 2.5 mg cause hypoglycemia in children 1-4 years old
  - 5 mg glyburide ingestion: Hypoglycemia reported in 79-year-old non-diabetic

Mechanism of Action
- Stimulates endogenous insulin secretion from beta islet cells in the pancreas

Clinical Manifestations
- Hypoglycemia
- Similar to insulin
- Potentially longer-acting in those with renal dysfunction (glyburide) and pediatrics
- Chlorpropamide associated with the syndrome of inappropriate antidiuretic hormone secretion and disulfiram reaction

Diagnostics
- Blood glucose q2hrs while awake, q1hr when asleep
- BMP
- Although sulfonylurea screens are available from reference laboratories they are not routinely needed.
  - Potentially useful in cases of undifferentiated recurrent hypoglycemia

Treatment
- Food/drink PO ad lib
- IV dextrose if hypoglycemic
  - D5W or D10W infusion titrated to maintain euglycemia
    - 0.5-1.0 g/kg, adjust based on size
  - If concentration > D12.5W central venous access needed
    - Adult: D50 (0.5 g/mL) IV
    - Pediatric: D25 (0.25 g/mL) IV
    - Neonates: D10 (0.1 g/mL) IV
  - Consider administering thiamine if deficient
- Octreotide
  - If hypoglycemia occurs
  - 1-2 mcg/kg SC, max 50 mcg q6hrs
  - Continuous infusion can be used

Disposition
- Admit
  - All intentional ingestions or unintentional in children
  - Severe, persistent, or worsening signs and symptoms or those requiring antidotal treatment

Thiazolidinediones

Sources
- Drugs used to treat diabetes (pioglitazone, rosiglitazone)

Toxic Dose
- Toxic dose undetermined

Mechanism of Action
- Increased insulin sensitivity, reduced glucose production in liver

Clinical Manifestations
- Hypoglycemia unlikely
- Hepatotoxicity with therapeutic use
- Fluid retention/CHF with therapeutic use
- Rosiglitazone linked to increase myocardial infarction with therapeutic use

Diagnostics
- Blood glucose q2hrs

Treatment
- Food/drink PO ad lib
- IV or oral dextrose if hypoglycemic
  - Oral glucose gel or tablets available while securing IV access
  - D5W or D10W infusion titrated to maintain euglycemia
    - 0.5-1.0 g/kg, adjust based on size
  - If concentration > D12.5W central venous access needed
    - Adult: D50 (0.5 g/mL) IV
    - Pediatric: D25 (0.25 g/mL) IV
    - Neonates: D10 (0.1 g/mL) IV
  - Goal to maintain glucose in normal range (70-110 mg/dL)

Disposition
- Observe minimum 6 hrs
- Admit severe, persistent, or worsening signs and symptoms

ANTIHISTAMINES & ANTIMUSCARINICS

Sources
- Antidysrhythmics (disopyramide, flecainide)
- Antipsychotics (clozapine, olanzapine, quetiapine)
- Antispasmodics
- Atropine
- Benztropine
- Cough and cold preparations
  - Chlorpheniramine
  - Diphenhydramine
  - Doxylamine
  - Hydroxyzine
- Glycopyrrolate
- Tricyclic antidepressants (TCAs)
- Plants
  - *Atropa bella-donna* (deadly nightshade, atropine derivative)
  - *Brugmansia* spp. (angel's trumpet)

- *Datura stramonium* (jimsonweed)
- *Hyoscyamus niger* (henbane, stinking nightshade)
- *Mandragora officinarum* (mandrake—but many other plants are also called mandrake)

Toxic Dose
- Antihistamine
  - Common estimate is 3-5x daily dose (diphenhydramine fatal at 20-40 mg/kg)

  PEARL. Second generation non-sedating (selective) H1-antagonists such as cetirizine, loratadine, and fexofenadine are less toxic

Mechanism of Action
- Antihistamine
  - Reversible, competitive inhibitors of H1 receptors
- Antimuscarinic
  - Competitively antagonizes peripheral and central muscarinic acetylcholine receptors

Clinical Manifestations (See Toxidrome Table, p. 282)

PEARL. "Red as a beet, dry as a bone, blind as a bat, mad as a hatter, hot as a hare, and full as a flask"

- Skin flushing
- Dry mouth/skin
- Mydriasis
- Delirium

  PEARL. Picking at nonexistent objects on bedsheets

  - Lilliputian type or Alice in Wonderland-like: perceiving people in different sizes
- Hyperthermia
- Urinary retention
- Constipation
- Sinus tachycardia

  PEARL. Tachycardia—one of earliest signs of peripheral anticholinergic toxicity but can be absent

  - Absence of tachycardia may be due to central antimuscarinic effects, non-significant ingestion, co-ingestion (β-blocker) or severe Na^+ channel blockade (QRS prolongation)

- Myoclonic jerking
- Seizures

PEARL. For some drugs precipitous fall in pH may result in worsening cardiotoxicity (TCAs; see Tricyclic Antidepressants, p. 136).

- QRS prolongation
  - Any substance that also blocks cardiac voltage-gated Na⁺ channels (diphenhydramine, hydroxyzine, TCAs, etc.)
- QT prolongation
  - Any substance that also blocks cardiac voltage-gated K⁺ channels (antipsychotics, diphenhydramine, TCAs, etc.)

Diagnostics
- Quantitative levels not available
- EKG
- CPK
- BMP

Treatment
- ABCDE
- Seizures
  - Diazepam
    - Adult: 5-10 mg IV q5min PRN
    - Pediatric: 0.2 mg/kg IV q5min, max 10 mg
  - Lorazepam
    - Adult: 2-4 mg IV q15min PRN
    - Pediatric: 0.1 mg/kg IV, max 4 mg
  - Repeat 0.1 mg/kg q15min
  - Phenobarbital, if benzodiazepines ineffective
    - 20 mg/kg IVPB
  - Propofol (if intubated)
    - 1-2 mg/kg IV bolus followed by continuous infusion 20 mcg/kg/min
- Delirium
  - Physostigmine
    - 2 mg IV over 5 min
    - Children: max 0.02 mg/kg IV over 5 min (max 0.5 mg)
    - Due to its short duration of action repeat dosing may be needed for recrudescence of agitation/delirium

> **PEARL.** Contraindications include, bradycardia, any cardiac conduction abnormalities, seizure, or history of seizure disorder, asthma or bronchospasm

- Consider administering dose of benzodiazepines in conjunction with physostigmine to raise seizure threshold
- Lower rates of intubations than benzodiazepines
- QRS prolongation and hypotension
  - Sodium bicarbonate
    - Bolus: 1-2 mEq/kg IVP over 1-2 min
    - Infusion: 100-150 mEq in 1 L D5W @ 150-200 mL/h (2x maintenance in pediatrics)
- QT prolongation
  - Electrolyte correction with replacement of Ca^{2+}, K^+, Mg^{2+}
- Hyperthermia: Aggressive cooling and control of agitation/motor activity
- Urinary retention: Indwelling urinary catheter

Disposition
- Observe minimum 6 hrs
- Admit severe, persistent, or worsening signs and symptoms or those requiring antidotal treatment

ANTIHYPERTENSIVES (ACE INHIBITORS, α2-AGONISTS, VASODILATORS)

ACE Inhibitors/ARB

Sources
- Ace inhibitors (medications ending in "pril")
- Angiotensin receptor blocker (ARBs)

Toxic Dose
- Wide therapeutic index and minimal toxicity, even up to 420 mg lisinopril

Mechanism of Action
- Blocks angiotensin I to II, which reduces vasoconstriction and aldosterone activity
- Bradykinin and endogenous enkephalins elevated
- Direct ARB

Clinical Manifestations
- Acute
  - Hypotension
  - Hyperkalemia
    - Especially in patients with renal insufficiency and concomitant use of nonsteroidal anti-inflammatory drugs and trimethoprim/sulfamethoxazole
- Chronic
  - Dry cough
- Angioedema
  - Generally occurs to tongue, lips, and face but can develop intestinal angioedema
    - Overall incidence is only approximately 0.1-0.7% but up to 5 times greater in patients of African descent
    - One-third of these reactions occur within hours of first dose and another third within the first week. Remaining one-third of cases can occur at any time during therapy, even after years
    - Rate of angioedema from ARBs is lower than from ACE inhibitors
    - Angioedema can wax and wane

Diagnostics
- No specific test
- BMP

Treatment
- ABCDE
- Hypotension
  - IVF
  - Vasopressor when unresponsive to IVF
- Angioedema
  - Several therapies are effective for hereditary angioedema that are not demonstrated to be effective for ACE inhibitor induced angioedema
    - C1 esterase concentrate
      - Any benefit may occur when administered in first few hours of symptom onset
    - Icatibant
      - Bradykinin B2-receptor antagonist
      - Largest randomized trial did not show superiority compared to placebo

- FFP
  - May degrade high concentrations of bradykinin and while there may be utility in hereditary angioedema, no definitive evidence that improves angioedema from ace inhibitors
- Steroids and antihistamines
  - Do not improve angioedema from ace inhibitors

Disposition
- Observe minimum 6 hrs
- Admit
  - Severe, persistent, or worsening signs and symptoms or those requiring antidotal treatment
  - Angioedema (or at least prolonged observation)

α-1 Antagonists

Sources
- Prazosin
- Terazosin
- Doxazosin

Toxic Doses
- Hypotension has been reported after 200 mg ingestion

Mechanism of action
- Peripheral α-1 antagonists directly relax smooth muscle

Clinical Manifestations
- Hypotension
- Orthostatic hypotension
- Syncope

Diagnostics
- No specific test
- Evaluate for other causes of syncope and hypotension
  - EKG
  - BMP
  - Pregnancy test

Treatment
- ABCDE
- Hypotension
  - IVF
  - Phenylephrine
    - Initiate 100-180 mcg /min, then titrate to goal MAP
  - Norepinephrine
    - Infusion: 0.05 mcg/kg/min, then titrate by 0.02 mcg/kg/min q5min to goal MAP
    - No true max and higher dosing may be required

Disposition
- Observe minimum 6 hrs
- Admit severe, persistent, or worsening signs and symptoms

α-2 Agonists

Sources
- Clonidine
  - Compounding creams
  - Tablets
  - Patches
- Guanfacine
- Guanabenz
- Imidazolines
- Methyldopa
- Tizanidine
- Dexmedetomidine

Toxic Dose
- Significant toxicity may occur with clonidine, particularly in children with ingestions as small as 0.1 mg
- 4 mg guanfacine ingestions in children have caused toxicity

Mechanism of Action
- Reduction of sympathetic outflow from CNS by stimulating presynaptic α-2-adrenergic receptors in the brain
- Prevents release of norepinephrine from presynaptic neuron
- Abrupt cessation may result in excessive sympathetic activity seen as rebound hypertension

PEARL. Large ingestions can temporarily stimulate postsynaptic α-2 adrenergic receptors resulting in transient hypertension

Clinical Manifestations
- CV
  - Hypertension
    - Often self-limited and short-lasting
    - Usually during intravenous administration or in moderate to large oral overdoses
  - Bradycardia or AV block
  - Hypotension (may be delayed, particularly in the patient who presents with hypertension)
- CNS
  - Decreased level of consciousness, often responsive to tactile stimulus
  - Miosis (may resemble opioid poisoning)
  - Hypothermia (may last several hours)
- Pulmonary
  - CNS depression may result in loss of protective airway reflexes but significant respiratory depression is uncommon

Diagnostics
- No specific test
- EKG

Treatment
- ABCDE
- Hypertension

    PEARL. Typically transient and does not require treatment

- Hypotension
  - IVF
  - Dopamine
    - Adult/pediatric: 5 mcg/kg/min IV, increase PRN 5-10 g/kg/min q10min to max 50 g/kg/min
  - Norepinephrine
    - As it is a direct vasopressor, may be preferred compared to dopamine
    - Infusion: 0.05 mcg/kg/min, then titrate by 0.02 mcg/kg/min q5min to goal MAP
  - Naloxone
    - Reversal of toxicity with naloxone is controversial. It is typically used when clinical manifestations of a-2 agonists are mistaken for opioid toxicity

- Bradycardia
  - Atropine
    - Adult: 0.5 mg q3-5min
    - Pediatric: 0.02 mg/kg IV (minimum dose 0.1 mg when > 5 kg, max doses 0.5 mg) q3-5min
  - Dopamine
    - Adult/pediatrics: 5 mcg/kg/min IV, increase PRN 5-10 g/kg/min q10min to max 50 g/kg/min
- Respiratory depression
  - Children may respond to tactile stimulation
  - Intubation or advanced airway placement is rarely required

Disposition
- Observe minimum 6 hrs (note: some sources recommend up to 12 hrs)
- Admit severe, persistent, or worsening signs and symptoms

β-Adrenergic Antagonists

Source
- Antihypertensive medications
- Ophthalmic drops

Mechanism of Action
- Antagonizes β receptors

PEARL. "Membrane Stabilizing" β-blockers (propranolol) inhibit fast Na$^+$ channels, causing QRS prolongation and seizures

PEARL. Sotalol will block K$^+$ efflux and increase QT, predisposing to torsades de pointes

Toxic Dose
- Response variable, but ingestions 2-3x therapeutic dose can cause toxicity, especially sustained-release preparations

Clinical Manifestations
- Dependent on dosage and specific medication
  - CV
    - Hypotension
    - Bradycardia
    - AV block
    - Heart failure
    - QRS prolongation (propranolol)
    - Torsades de pointes (sotalol)

- Pulmonary
  - Bronchospasm
- Metabolic
  - Hypoglycemia (more common in pediatrics)
  - Hyperkalemia

  PEARL. Low blood sugar may help differentiate from Ca^{2+} blocker toxicity

- CNS
  - Usually secondary to cerebral hypoperfusion
  - Except propranolol, which crosses blood-brain barrier
  - Mentation may be maintained initially until cardiovascular toxicity becomes severe
  - Somnolence
  - Coma
  - Seizures (propranolol)

Diagnostics
- EKG
- ECHO
- BMP
- Troponin
- CPK
- CXR
- ABG

Treatment
- ABCDE
- GI decontamination (charcoal, GI lavage) may be considered for large or life-threatening ingestions with expert consultation
- Atropine
  - Adult: 0.5 mg q3-5min
  - Pediatric: 0.02 mg/kg IV (minimum dose 0.1 mg when > 5 kg, max doses 0.5 mg) q3-5min
  - Effect may be minimal or transient
- Glucagon
  - Adult: 50 mcg/kg (typically start with 3-5 mg; max 10 mg) IV over 1-2 min, repeat q10-15min 1-2 times PRN; higher doses may be necessary if initial bolus ineffective
  - Then: start infusion at effective bolus dose, typically 2-5 mg/h (max 10 mg/h) IV in D5W
  - Pediatric: 50 mcg/kg IV load, then 70 mcg/kg/hr
    - Dose escalation may be limited by vomiting

- Vasopressors
    - Epinephrine
        - Infusion: Initial 0.05-2 mcg/kg/min. Titrate by 0.02-0.05 mcg/kg/min q15min to goal MAP
        - No true max and higher dosing may be required
    - Norepinephrine
        - Infusion: 0.05 mcg/kg/min, then titrate by 0.02 mcg/kg/min q5min to goal MAP
        - No true max and higher dosing may be required
    - Vasopressin
        - 0.01 U/min titrate to goal MAP
    - Phenylephrine
        - Initiate 100-180 mcg/min, then titrate to goal MAP
- High dose insulin
    - Insulin: 1 U/kg IV bolus
    - Then: 0.5-1.0 U/kg/hr IV drip
        - Increase if no effect in 15 min
        - Titrate up to 10 U/kg/hr
        - Check capillary glucose q30min initially & titrated to maintain euglycemia
    - Dextrose: ± 25-50 g (0.5-1 g/kg) IV bolus (unless glucose > 300 mg/dL)
    - Then: 0.25-0.5 g/kg/h IV drip
- Cardiac pacing
    - 50-60
- ECMO
    - If above methods fail/refractory shock
- ILE
    - If above methods fail/refractory shock
    - Loading dose 1.5 mL/kg 20% solution over 1 min
        - May repeat for persistent dysrhythmias
    - Infusion: 0.25 mL/kg/min over 30-60 min
- QRS prolongation and hypotension
    - Sodium bicarbonate
        - Bolus: 1-2 mEq/kg IVP over 1-2 min, repeat until QRS narrows or limited by sodium > 155 or pH > 7.55
        - Infusion: 100-150 mEq in 1 L D5W @ 150-200 mL/h (2x maintenance in pediatrics)

Disposition
- Immediate release formulation: Observe minimum 6 hrs
- Admit severe, persistent, or worsening signs and symptoms or those requiring antidotal treatment

Calcium Channel Antagonists

Source
- Dihydropyridine (DHP): Amlodipine
- Phenylalkylamines (Non-DHP): Verapamil
- Benzothiazepines (Non-DHP): Diltiazem

Toxic Dose
- Low toxic-therapeutic ratio and any dose outside of therapeutic range—especially sustained release preparations—can be associated with toxicity

Mechanism of Action
- Inhibits Ca^{2+} entry through maintaining voltage gated L-type channels in closed state
  — DHPs have higher affinity for L-type Ca^{2+} channels in vasculature
  — Non-DHPs have higher affinity for cardiac L-type Ca^{2+} channels
  — Above specificity lost in overdose
- Block Ca^{2+} mediated insulin release by pancreatic B-Islet cells

PEARL. Dihydropyridine toxicity may cause reflex tachycardia

Clinical Manifestations
- Dependent on dosage and specific medication
  — CV
    - Hypotension
      - Peripheral vasodilatation (predominates in DHP toxicity)
      - Myocardial depression (and vasodilation seen in Non-DHP toxicity)
    - Bradycardia
    - AV conduction abnormalities
    - Cardiogenic shock
    - Syncope
  — Metabolic/GI
    - Hyperglycemia

PEARL. Elevated glucose may help differentiate from β-blocker toxicity and may correlate with severity of toxicity

PEARL. Abdominal pain may be a sign of mesenteric ischemia
- CNS
  - CNS depression/ altered mentation
    - Secondary to hypoperfusion and metabolic derangements or coingestants

Diagnostics
- EKG
- ECHO
- BMP
- Troponin
- CPK
- CXR
- ABG

Treatment
- ABCDE
- Gastric decontamination
  - Consider for large ingestion if not contraindicated
- Bradycardia/hypotension
  - Atropine
    - Adult: 0.5 mg q3-5min
    - Pediatric: 0.02 mg/kg IV (minimum dose 0.1 mg when > 5 kg, max doses 0.5 mg) q3-5min
    - Effect likely transient or minimal
  - Cardiac pacing
    - 50-60 bpm
  - Calcium
    - Adult: CaCl 10% 1 g IV over 10-15 min (central line only) or CaGluconate 10% 3 g IV over 5-10 min if no central access
    - Pediatric: CaCl 10% 20 mg/kg IV over 10-15 min (central line only) or CaGluconate 10% 60-100 mg/kg IV over 5-10 min if no central access, not to exceed adult dose
  - Glucagon
    - Adult: 50 mcg/kg (typically start with 3-5 mg; max 10 mg) IV over 1-2 min, repeat q10-15min 1-2 times PRN; higher doses may be necessary if initial bolus ineffective
    - Then: 2-5 mg/h (max 10 mg/h) IV in D5W
    - Pediatric: 50 mcg/kg IV load, then 70 mcg/kg/hr
      - Vomiting may occur

- Vasopressors
  - Epinephrine
    - Infusion: Initial 0.05-2 mcg/kg/min. Titrate by 0.02-0.05 mcg/kg/min q15min to goal MAP
    - No true max and higher dosing may be required
  - Norepinephrine
    - Infusion: 0.05 mcg/kg/min, then titrate by 0.02 mcg/kg/min q5min to goal MAP
    - No true max and higher dosing may be required
  - Vasopressin
    - 0.01 U/min titrate to goal MAP
  - Phenylephrine
    - Initiate 100-180 mcg /min, then titrate to goal MAP
- High dose insulin
  - Insulin: 1 U/kg IV bolus
  - Then: 0.5-1.0 U/kg/hr IV drip
    - Increase if no effect in 15 min
    - Titrate up to 10 U/kg/hr
    - Check capillary glucose q30min initially & titrated to maintain euglycemia
  - Dextrose: ± 25-50 g (0.5-1 g/kg) IV bolus (unless glucose > 300 mg/dL)
  - *Then*: 0.25-0.5 g/kg/h IV drip
- ECMO
  - If prior methods fail/refractory shock
- ILE
  - If prior methods fail/refractory shock
  - Loading dose 1.5 mL/kg 20% solution over 1 min
  - May repeat for persistent dysrhythmias
    - Infusion: 0.25 mL/kg/min over 30-60 min

Disposition

- Immediate release formulation: Observe minimum 6 hrs
- Admit
  - All patients with extended release preparation ingestions or unintentional in children
  - Severe, persistent, or worsening signs and symptoms or those requiring antidotal treatment

Diuretics

Sources
- Furosemide
- Hydrochlorothiazide
- Spironolactone

Toxic Doses
- Significant toxicity unlikely if ingestion < typical daily dose

Clinical Manifestations
- CV
  - Hypotension
- Metabolic
  - Hyponatremia
    - Vomiting, seizures, altered mental status
  - Hypokalemia
    - Ventricular arrhythmias
  - Hyperkalemia
    - Spironolactone
    - Ventricular arrhythmias
  - Hypercalcemia
    - Thiazide diuretics

Diagnostics
- BMP

Treatment
- ABCDE
- Hypotension: IVF
- Electrolyte repletion

Disposition
- Observe minimum 6 hrs
- Admit severe, persistent, or worsening signs or symptoms

Vasodilators

Sources
- Hydralazine
- Minoxidil
- Nitroglycerin
- Nitroprusside

Toxic Doses
- Hydralazine: Highest known dose survived: 10 g orally in adults
- Minoxidil: Toxicity reported after 1.3 g ingestion of topical solution

Mechanism of Action
- Dilate smooth muscle via nitric oxide

Clinical Manifestations
- Hypotension
- Reflex tachycardia
- Nitroprusside
  - Endogenously releases cyanide which is detoxified to form thiocyanate
  - Nitroprusside is coformulated with thiosulfate to prevent cyanide toxicity
  - Thiocyanate toxicity is seen with prolonged infusions, high doses, renal insufficiency
    - Abdominal pain
    - Vomiting
    - CNS dysfunction (confusion, agitation)
  - Inadequate thiosulfate can result in cyanide poisoning
  (See antidote, p. 272)
    - Lethargy, confusion, coma, seizures
    - Hypotension
    - Tachycardia
    - Lactic acidosis
- Hydralazine
  - Vasculitis
  - Hemolytic anemia

Diagnostics
- Nitroprusside
  - Whole blood cyanide concentration
    - Difficult to interpret often falsely elevated
    - Does not return in a clinically useful timeframe
    - Red blood cell cyanide concentrations would be more accurate
  - Thiocyanate concentration can be obtained for suspected thiocyanate toxicity; results unlikely to return in clinically useful timeframe
  - Lactate
  - ABG, VBG

Treatment
- ABCDE
- Hypotension
  - Stop infusion
  - IVF
  - Norepinephrine
    - Infusion: 0.05 mcg/kg/min, then titrate by 0.02 mcg/kg/min q5min to goal MAP
    - No true max and higher dosing may be required
  - Phenylephrine: Initiate 100-180 mcg /min, then titrate to goal MAP
  - ECMO: Consider for refractory hypotension
- Cyanide
  - Hydroxocobalamin
    - Adult: 5g IV, may repeat × 1
    - Pediatric: 70 mg/kg (max 5 g) IV over 30 min
  - Sodium thiosulfate, sodium nitrite
- Thiocyanate: HD

Disposition
- Observe minimum 6 hrs
- Admit severe, persistent, or worsening signs and symptoms or those requiring antidotal treatment

ANTIPSYCHOTICS

Typical Antipsychotics

Sources
- Chlorpromazine
- Chlorprothixene
- Droperidol
- Fluphenazine
- Haloperidol
- Pimozide
- Promethazine
- Thioridazine
- Trifluoperazine

Toxic Dose
- Variable; tolerance to sedative effects by chronic users

Mechanism of Action
- D_2 antagonism considered therapeutic mechanism of action
- Other effects
  - Fast Na^+ channel blockade
  - Delayed rectifier K^+ channel blockade
  - α1-antagonism
  - Muscarinic antagonism

Clinical Manifestations
- CNS
  - Extrapyramidal syndromes (akathisia, dystonia, parkinsonism, tardive dyskinesia)
    - May also see with therapeutic dosing
  - Somnolence
  - Seizures
  - Anticholinergic toxidrome (See Toxidrome Table, p. 282)
    - Phenothiazines
    - Agents that do not have anti-muscarinic activity: haloperidol, fluphenazine, perphenazine, trifluoperazine, pimozide
  - Hyperthermia
- CV
  - Hypotension
  - Tachycardia
  - QRS prolongation
  - QT prolongation

  PEARL. Thioridazine is the most cardiotoxic typical antipsychotic and is associated with greatest QT prolongation

- Neuroleptic Malignant Syndrome (See NMS, p. 245)
  - Hyperthermia
  - Muscular rigidity
  - Altered mental status
  - Autonomic instability

Diagnostics
- EKG
- BMP
- CPK, other exclusionary workup for NMS (r/o infection, etc.)

Treatment
- ABCDE
- Anticholinergic Delirium
  - Titration of benzodiazepines, supportive care, indwelling catheter for urinary retention, cooling
  - Physostigmine
    - Contraindicated in patients with asthma or history of bronchospasm, bradycardia or cardiac conduction abnormalities, seizures
    - Expect recrudescence of signs of anticholinergic toxicity due short duration of action
      - Adult: 0.5-1 mg IV over > 5 min; may repeat in 5-10 min PRN × 1-2 doses (maximum total dose of 2 mg in 1 hr)
      - Pediatric: 0.02 mg/kg (max 0.5 mg) as above Indication: Severe anticholinergic toxicity
- Hypotension
  - IVF 0.9% sodium chloride 30-40 mL/kg
    - Norepinephrine
      - Infusion: 0.05 mcg/kg/min, then titrate by 0.02 mcg/kg/min q5min to goal MAP
      - No true max and higher dosing may be required
- EKG changes
  - QRS prolongation (+t40 aVR)
    - Sodium bicarbonate
      - Bolus: 1-2 mEq/kg IVP over 1-2 min, with continuous rhythm strip running
      - Infusion: 100-150 mEq in 1 L D5W @ 150-200 mL/h (2x maintenance)
      - Caution if QT prolongation present as sodium bicarbonate administration may worsen it
  - QT prolongation
  - Correct electrolytes abnormalities (K^+, Mg^{2+}, Ca^{2+})
- NMS (See p. 245)
  - Cooling
  - Benzodiazepines
  - Paralysis
- Seizures
  - Diazepam
    - Adult: 5-10 mg IV q5 mins PRN
    - Pediatric: 0.2 mg/kg IV q5min, max 10 mg

- Lorazepam
  - Adult: 2-4 mg IV q15 mins PRN
  - Pediatric: 0.1 mg/kg IV, max 4 mg
    - Repeat 0.1 mg/kg q 15 mins
- Phenobarbital, if benzodiazepines ineffective
  - 20 mg/kg IVPB
- Propofol (if intubated)
  - 1-2 mg/kg IV bolus followed by continuous infusion 20 mcg/kg/min

Disposition
- Observe minimum 6 hrs
- Admit severe, persistent, or worsening signs and symptoms

Atypical Antipsychotics

Sources
- Most common medications
  - Risperidone
  - Quetiapine
  - Clozapine
  - Aripiprazole
  - Olanzapine
  - Ziprasidone

Toxic Doses
- Highly variable and tolerance to medications is well-described

(that's the buller for Toxic Doses)

Mechanism of Action
- D2 antagonism (less than seen with typical antipsychotics)
- Treat both positive and negative symptoms of schizophrenia
- Antagonism at other receptors with varying affinities
  - Serotonin (5HT-2A)
  - Muscarinic (m_1)
  - Histamine (H_1)
  - α-adrenergic ($α_1$)
  - Cardiac fast Na⁺ channels (I_{NA})
  - Cardiac delayed rectifier potassium channels (I_K)

Clinical Manifestations
- ACUTE toxicity
  - Clinical effects may be predicted by the agent's unique receptor binding profile
    - CNS depression
      - Quetiapine is being abused due to its CNS effects
    - Anticholinergic toxicity

      PEARL. Clozapine associated with salivation (activates M4 receptor) but still can cause anticholinergic toxicity

      PEARL. Atypicals with α-adrenergic antagonism may cause miosis (olanzapine, clozapine, quetiapine)

    - Hypotension
    - Tachycardia
    - QT prolongation

      PEARL. Ziprasidone can significantly prolong the QT

    - Extrapyramidal symptoms
    - Seizures

      PEARL. Quetiapine can cause seizures

- CHRONIC toxicity
  - Extrapyramidal symptoms
  - NMS
    - Symptoms may develop over 2-10 days. Gradual onset as compared to serotonin syndrome
      - Muscular rigidity (lead pipe)
      - Hyperthermia
      - Rhabdomyolysis
      - Autonomic dysfunction (including diaphoresis)
      - Altered mental status
  - Clozapine
    - Agranulocytosis
    - Myocarditis/cardiomyopathy
  - Diabetes (metabolic syndrome)

Diagnostics
- Specific concentrations not readily available
- EKG
- CBC
- CPK
- BMP

Treatment
- ABCDE
- Anticholinergic delirium
- QRS prolongation
    - Sodium bicarbonate or sodium acetate
        - 100-150 mEq in 1 liter of D5W at 1.5 maintenance. Can also administer sodium bicarbonate as a bolus. Sodium acetate cannot be administered as a bolus
- QT prolongation
    - Correct electrolyte disturbance
- EPS symptoms-may reoccur over multiple days
    - Diphenhydramine/benztropine
    - Benzodiazepines
- NMS (See p. 245)

Disposition
- Observe minimum 6 hrs
- Admit
    - Severe, persistent, or worsening signs or symptoms
    - NMS

DIGOXIN

Sources
- Pharmaceuticals
- Non-pharmaceutical/natural sources
    - Oleander
    - Lily of the valley
    - Red squill
    - Foxglove
    - *Bufo* spp. (toad) derived
        - Cane toad, Colorado River toad
        - Aphrodisiac—"Love Stone", "Ch'an Su"

Toxic Dose
- Acute: ingestion 1 mg in a child or 3 mg in adult can result in serum concentrations well above therapeutic range; supratherapeutic concentration

Mechanism of Action

PEARL. Inhibits Na/K-ATPase

- Increased intracellular calcium results in positive inotropy, chronotropy, and increased automaticity

PEARL. Increased vagal tone leading to slowed conduction through SA/AV nodes resulting in bradycardia and heart blocks

Clinical Manifestations
- CV
  - PVCs and PACs
  - Bradydysrhythmias: sinus brady, AFib (or any atrial tachycardia) with slow ventricular response, heart blocks
  - Ventricular dysrhythmias: VTach, VFib, bidirectional VTach
- Other
  - Acute
    - N/V
    - Hyperkalemia
  - Chronic
    - Altered mental status
    - N/V
    - Chromatopsia (yellow halo around lights): very rare
    - Renal dysfunction: impaired digoxin clearance

PEARL. ACUTE and CHRONIC clinical findings can overlap

Diagnostics
- Serum digoxin concentration
  - 2 ng/mL (although toxicity may occur at lower concentrations)
  - Therapeutic range: 0.5-0.8 ng/mL
    - Interpret based on time since ingestion/last dose (> 6 hours for post-distribution)

PEARL. Concentrations drawn < **6 hrs** from last dose are pre-distribution that may be elevated and not reflective of tissue burden

PEARL. Clinical manifestations of toxicity are more important than serum concentrations; serum digoxin concentration does not correlate with severity of non-pharmaceutical sources of toxicity and should not be used to dose digoxin immune FAB

PEARL. Endogenous digoxin-like substances (EDLS) can cross-react with serum digoxin concentration in absence of actual digoxin exposure

  - Hepatic failure
  - Renal failure
  - Pregnancy
  - CHF

- Potassium
  - ACUTE toxicity: Hyperkalemia (> 5.0 mEq/L) serves as a predictor of mortality
  - CHRONIC toxicity
    - Hypokalemia: May worsen toxicity, typically from co-administration of medications that lower potassium (diuretics)
    - Hyperkalemia: May occur with concomitant renal failure
    - Hypomagnesemia
- EKG
  - Ectopy: PVCs, PACs, delayed afterdepolarizations
    - Most common finding
  - Bidirectional VT
    - Although not pathognomonic, highly suggestive of digoxin toxicity
  - SVT with slow ventricular response

    PEARL. Never see supraventricular dysrhythmia with rapid ventricular response

  - Prolonged PR
  - Shortened QT
  - Bradydysrhythmia
  - AV block
  - ST/T-wave scooping seen in therapeutic use; not indicative of toxicity
  - Renal function

Treatment

- ABCDE
- Digoxin immune FAB
  - Life-threatening dysrhythmias or hemodynamic instability
  - Hyperkalemia
    - ACUTE toxicity: K^+ > 5.0 mEq/L
    - Some sources recommend empiric treatment for:
      - Adult: 10 mg ingestion
      - Pediatric: 4 mg ingestion
      - Consider in serum concentration > 15 ng/mL within 6 hrs of ingestion
      - Serum concentration > 10 ng/mL steady state
  - ACUTE toxicity
    - Known serum digoxin concentration
      - Dose (in vials) = (serum digoxin [ng/mL] × weight in kg)/100
    - Unknown digoxin amount with toxicity
      - Total dose: 10 vials

- Known amount of digoxin ingested with toxicity, concentration unavailable
  - Dose (in vials) = Total mg digoxin ingested × 2
  - 1 vial binds 0.5 mg digoxin
- CHRONIC toxicity
  - For known serum digoxin concentration
    - Dose (in vials) = (serum digoxin [ng/mL] × weight in kg) / 100
  - In absence of serum digoxin concentration: 3-6 vials

  PEARL. After treatment with digoxin immune FAB, only free digoxin concentrations can be used to guide treatment; DO NOT USE total serum concentrations as they are falsely elevated

  - Electrolyte abnormalities
    - Hyperkalemia
      - Serum K^+ concentration will fall after digoxin immune FAB administration
      - Temporizing efforts with insulin, dextrose, sodium bicarbonate should be used judiciously
      - Digoxin toxicity produces intracellular hypercalcemia, avoiding administration of calcium may be prudent
- Hypokalemia/hypomagnesemia
  - May occur with CHRONIC toxicity and exacerbate toxicity
  - Judicious electrolyte replacement
    - Dysrhythmias
      - Digoxin immune FAB: primary therapy; other therapies in setting of digoxin-induced dysrhythmias often ineffective
        - Ingestion known: # vials = (amount mg × 0.8) / 0.5 mg
        - Concentration known: # vials = [concentration (ng/mL) × weight in kg] / 100
        - Unknown ingestion/concentration: Empiric therapy
        - Adult: 10 vials (acute); 3-6 vials (chronic)
        - Pediatric: 1-2 vials
    - Lidocaine: tachyarrhythmias
      - Adult: 1-1.5 mg/kg IV ×1 over 2 min; repeat 0.5 to 0.75 mg/kg bolus q5-10min (max cumulative dose 3 mg/kg). Follow by infusion = 1-4 mg/min; titrate by 1-2 mg/min q10min. After 24 hrs continuous infusion, decrease infusion rate by 50%. Reduce dose in patients with CHF, shock, or hepatic disease. Max = 4 mg/min
      - Pediatric: 1 mg/kg/dose; follow with continuous IV infusion 20-50 mcg/kg/minute. May administer second bolus if delay between initial bolus and start of infusion is > 15 min. Do not exceed 20 mcg/kg/min in patients with shock, hepatic disease, cardiac arrest, or CHF

- Atropine: bradycardia and heart block
  - Adult: 0.5 mg q3-5min
  - Pediatric: 0.02 mg/kg IV (minimum dose 0.1 mg when > 5 kg, max doses 0.5 mg) q3-5min
- Cardioversion for unstable VT or defibrillation for VF

PEARL. Avoid amiodarone, procainamide, β-blockers, calcium channel blockers, intravenous pacing—may increase ventricular arrhythmias/AV block

PEARL. Hemodialysis is ineffective in removing cardiac glycosides

Disposition
- Acute ingestion
  - Observe minimum 6 hrs
  - Admit severe, persistent, or worsening signs and symptoms or those requiring antidotal treatment
- Chronic toxicity
  - Admit for continuous cardiac monitoring, serial digoxin concentrations, and EKGs
  - Evaluate for underlying cause of digoxin toxicity

METHOTREXATE

Source
- Medications for rheumatologic conditions, chemotherapeutic, abortifacient

Toxic Dose
- Therapeutic doses vary widely
  - Rheumatology (RA, psoriasis): Up to 30 mg/week in adults; up to 10 mg/m2/week in children (JIA)
  - Ectopic pregnancy: Typically 50 mg/m2; can be repeated
  - Neoplastic disease: High-dose MTX is ≥ 500 mg/m2 IV, used with leucovorin rescue
  - Intrathecal: Variable, but typically up to 15 mg
- Toxic doses vary depending on route and chronicity
  - Intrathecal injection > 500 mg associated with severe morbidity or death
  - Toxicity occurs after prolonged use (> 2 years) or after total oral dose of 1.5 g

Mechanism of Action
- Folic acid antagonist that inhibits dihydrofolate reductase; interferes with DNA synthesis

Clinical Manifestations

PEARL. ACUTE, oral ingestions largely benign and asymptomatic; toxicity from infusion or intrathecal administration

- GI
  - N/V/D
  - Ulcerative stomatitis
  - Elevated LFT
- Heme
  - Bone marrow suppression
- CNS
  - Seizure
  - Coma
- Renal
  - Acute tubular necrosis
- Derm
  - Toxic epidermal necrolysis
  - Stevens-Johnson syndrome
  - Exfoliative dermatitis
  - Erythema multiforme

Diagnostics

- Serum methotrexate concentration
  - Toxic > 1 mcmol/L at 48 hrs
- CBC
- BMP
- LFT
- UA

Treatment

- ABCDE
- IV hydration
- Urine alkalinization
- Leucovorin
  - For IV MTX overdose, use pharmacokinetically-guided rescue nomogram for leucovorin dosing, or 100 mg/m2 IV over 15-30 mins (max 160 mg/min) q3-6hrs
  - Treatment duration depends on MTX concentration and clinical effect
  - For PO MTX overdose:
    - Dose 1:1 based on estimated absorbed dose
    - Most acute oral overdoses would not need leucovorin due to the limited bioavailability with high doses

- Glucarpidase 50 units/kg IV
  - Bone marrow suppression also consider granulocyte-stimulating factor, RBC, and/or platelet transfusion
- Intrathecal toxicity
  - IV leucovorin as above
  - Consider CSF drainage via lumbar puncture, CSF exchange, or ventriculo-lumbar perfusion
  - IV dexamethasone: 4 mg q6hrs × 4 doses

PEARL. Intrathecal glucarpidase (carboxypeptidase): 2000 units over 5 min

Disposition
- Discharge oral ingestion without evidence of effect or systemic toxicity
- Admit severe, persistent, or worsening signs and symptoms or those requiring antidotal treatment

METHYLXANTHINES

Sources
- Caffeine
- Theophylline
- Theobromine

Toxic Dose
- Caffeine PO
  - \> 20 mg/kg
    - Restlessness
    - Insomnia
  - \> 150-200 mg/kg life-threatening
- Theophylline PO
  - \> 50 mg/kg

Mechanism of Action
- Increased endogenous release of catecholamines producing β1 and β2 agonism
- Inhibits phosphodiesterase, resulting in elevated cAMP = smooth muscle relaxation, peripheral vasodilation, myocardial stimulation, CNS excitation
- Adenosine antagonism

Clinical Manifestations
- GI
  - N/V more common in acute OD, often difficult to control
  - Gastritis more common in chronic use
- CV
  - Atrial and ventricular tachydysrhythmias
  - Myocardial ischemia/infarction
  - Widened pulse pressure
  - Hypotension (vasodilation)
  - Cerebral vasoconstriction
  - Renal vasodilation (increased diuresis)
- Metabolic

  PEARL. Hypokalemia (because of shift, not total loss of K$^+$)

  - Hypomagnesemia
  - Hypophosphatemia
  - Hyperglycemia
  - Lactemia
  - Metabolic acidosis
  - Hyperthermia
- CNS
  - Anxiety
  - Agitation
  - Tremor
  - Seizures
- Musculoskeletal
  - Myoclonus, hypertonicity, rhabdomyolysis
- Pulmonary
  - Tachypnea/hyperventilation resulting in respiratory alkalosis

Diagnostics
- Serum caffeine concentration (not typically attainable at many hospital labs)
  - > 80 mcg/mL: life-threatening
- Serum theophylline concentration
  - > 40 mcg/mL: life-threatening in setting of chronic toxicity
  - > 80 mcg/mL life-threatening in setting of acute toxicity
  - Delayed peak plasma concentration with sustained release formulations
- EKG
- CPK
- ABG/VBG
- BMP

Treatment

- ABCDE
  - GI decontamination should be considered because of life-threatening nature of toxicity but can be technically difficult due to refractory vomiting
  - Consider multiple-dose activated charcoal if vomiting controlled
    - 1 g/kg PO initially, then reassess to determine if repeat dose can be administered with goal of q4-6hrs × 4 doses
  - Consider whole bowel irrigation if vomiting controlled and sustained-release theophylline
- Seizures and CNS excitation
  - Diazepam
    - Adult: 5-10 mg IV q5-10min PRN
    - Pediatric: 0.15-0.2 mg/kg IV q5-10min
  - Lorazepam
    - Adult: 2-4 mg IV q10-15min PRN
    - Pediatric 0.1 mg/kg IV q10-15min
  - Phenobarbital (if refractory to benzodiazepines)
    - 20 mg/kg IV (anticonvulsant dose; secure airway likely needed)
  - Propofol (if intubated)
    - Continuous infusion of 5 mcg/kg/min titrate (rec. max of 55 mcg/kg/min)
- Hypotension/shock and cardiac toxicity
  - Fluid resuscitation
  - Vasopressor with prominent α1 agonist activity (phenylephrine, norepinephrine)
  - Although β-blockers are recommended by some texts in cases of refractory shock this intervention should be used with caution and is contraindicated in patients with history of asthma or bronchospasm
  - Esmolol has short duration of action and β1 selectivity
  - Supraventricular tachydysrhythmias
  - Titration of benzodiazepines is first line therapy

PEARL. SVT from methylxanthine toxicity is often refractory to adenosine and if response is obtained it is typically short-lived

  - Consider diltiazem infusion
- Hypokalemia

PEARL. Cautious repletion because represents a shift, not absolute loss

- HD
  - Acute theophylline concentration
    - \> 90 mcg/mL and any sign

- Chronic theophylline concentration
  - \> 40 mcg/mL and either seizures, hypotension unresponsive to fluids, ventricular dysrhythmia

Disposition
- Admit
  - Severe, persistent, or worsening signs and symptoms
  - Intentional extended release theophylline ingestions

OPIOIDS

Sources
- Opioids: Produce an opium like effect or bind to an opioid receptor
  - Opiates are derived from the opium poppy
    - Morphine
    - Codeine (metabolized to morphine by CYP2D6)
    - Thebaine
  - Synthetic: Not derived from an opiate but causes opiate-like effects or binds to opioid receptors
    - Fentanyl
      - Analogs (sufentanil, carfentanil)
    - U-4770 (research chemical)
    - W-18 (research chemical)
    - Methadone
    - Meperidine
    - Tramadol (See subsection)
    - Loperamide (See subsection)
  - Semi-synthetic: Created by chemical modification of an opiate
    - Buprenorphine
    - Heroin
    - Hydrocodone
    - Hydromorphone
    - Oxycodone
    - Dextromethorphan
    - Oxymorphone

Mechanism of Action
- Agonize opiate (μ) receptors in central nervous, cardiovascular, pulmonary, and GI systems
  - Some opioids also bind other receptors including K and Δ receptors

Clinical Manifestations

- Mild/moderate overdose
  - Lethargy
  - Miotic "pinpoint" pupils
    - Dextromethorphan, propoxyphene, and meperidine may cause mydriasis
    - Additionally if opioid is combined with sympathomimetic agent (speedball) the patient may have mydriasis
  - Hypotension
  - Bradycardia
  - Diminished bowel sounds
  - Flaccid muscles
- Severe overdose
  - Decreased level of consciousness/coma
  - Respiratory depression
  - Non-cardiogenic pulmonary edema (exact etiology unknown)
  - Apnea
  - Sudden death
- Opioid withdrawal syndrome
  - Anxiety
  - Piloerection
  - Hyperesthesia
  - N/V/D
  - Yawning
  - Insomnia

PEARL. Sensorium preserved

PEARL. Neonates born to an opioid-dependent mother may be at risk of neonatal abstinence syndrome, which can cause seizures

PEARL. There are case reports of acute delirium being precipitated in patients receiving naltrexone while still having opioids in their system

- Methadone
  - QT prolongation
  - Strong consideration to admit for observation after overdose or if required naloxone
- Meperidine, tramadol, tapentadol
  - Seizures
- Meperidine, tramadol
  - Serotonin syndrome (See Serotonin Syndrome, p. 247)

- Hearing loss
  - Sensorineural hearing loss
  - Can occur with any opioid
  - Many will recover with abstinence but not all
- Fentanyl
  - Rigid chest
    - May be related to rapid IV push
    - Generally responds to naloxone
- Diphenoxylate and atropine
  - Diphenoxylate has limited GI absorption and works as an antidiarrheal agent by binding to local GI μ receptors
  - May result in systemic toxicity in children. Delayed or prolonged effects may occur due to combination of opioid and anticholinergic effects (from atropine) and a long acting metabolite of diphenoxylate
  - Prolonged observation/admission required because of delayed onset of symptoms after ingestions
- Loperamide (see subsection)
- Body packers
  - Internal concealment of meticulously sealed packages of illicit drugs with purpose of trafficking
  - Typically, in large quantities and may be a single type of drug
  - May take constipating agents to slow GI tract
  - If has respiratory depression, will need naloxone infusion and admission
  - Generally, does not require laparotomy unless concern for sympathomimetic agent
  - Can administer activated charcoal, whole bowel irrigation
  - Imaging, including CT, is not always accurate in identifying all packages but can be performed
- Body stuffers
  - Ingestion of loosely packaged bags of illicit drugs, usually just before being apprehended by law enforcement
  - May swallow or place in rectum or vagina
  - Fentanyl patch
    - Large amount of fentanyl remains even after patch has already been used
    - Chewed can have immediate effects
    - If rectal or placed on skin or swallowed intact, may have delayed effects
- Non-cardiogenic pulmonary edema
  - Underlying cause, whether direct effect of an opioid, naloxone, negative intrathoracic pressure, remains unclear

Diagnostics

> **PEARL.** Clinical diagnosis
> — Coma
> — Pinpoint pupils
> — Respiratory depression

- Awakening after administration of naloxone
  - If using as a determination that patient's AMS is from an opioid, ensure a true response to naloxone is observed. Other diagnoses have been missed as patients were thought to have some response to naloxone when it was coincidental
- Acetaminophen concentration (combination preparations common)
- Urine drug screen immunoassay detects morphine metabolites such as codeine, morphine, heroin
  - Typical ELISA screen tests for morphine
  - Semi/synthetics not routinely detected
  - Screen has a cutoff so can have a false negative if the concentration of the drug is very low
  - For other opioids, will either need to use drug specific ELISA screen (specific screen for methadone) or a form of gas chromatography/mass spectrometry
- Radiographs
  - Body packers: CT
    - 30-50% sensitivity, 100% PPV
    - Limited utility even with a large number of concealed packets
  - Body stuffers/fentanyl ingestion: Unreliable

Treatment

- ABCDE
- Standard PPE
- Respiratory depression: hypoxemia/hypercarbia
  - Naloxone
    - Adult: Start at 0.04-0.4 mg IV/IM/IN/IO; repeat dose if initial response not adequate and titrate up to max 10 mg. Titrate to RR ≥ 12 and sufficient tidal volume
      - If opioid naïve, can start with dose > 0.4 mg as less likely to precipitate opioid withdrawal
    - For reversal of intoxication from a novel opioid (fentanyl derivative) effective dose of naloxone is not known; some have suggested larger doses may be needed
      - Pediatric: 0.04-0.4 mg IV (IM, SQ, IO) and titrate to effect
      - If opioid naïve, can administer larger dosages as less likely to precipitate withdrawal

- Neonate: (asphyxia neonatorum) can administer via umbilical vein or IM or SQ at similar doses if cannot obtain an IV
- Continuous infusion for recurrent respiratory depression start infusion: 2/3 of reversal dose infused hourly
- Can precipitate acute withdrawal symptoms; use lowest dose necessary

PEARL. Naloxone duration of action is commonly shorter than many opioids so opioid toxicity can recur; continuous pulse oximeter and capnography encouraged

PEARL. Remember mainstay of therapy is airway protection, oxygenation, and ventilation

- If patients have respiratory failure or cardiopulmonary arrest naloxone should not delay definitive treatment

- Body packers
  - Activated charcoal
  - WBI: 1-2 liters/hr PEG via NGT to clear rectal effluent
  - Naloxone infusion
  - Surgical consult
    - Generally if only concealing opioids, surgery is not necessary unless obstructed
    - For sympathomimetic agent, exploratory laparotomy to remove remaining packets for signs of sympathomimetic toxicity or obstruction
- Constipation
  - Methylnaltrexone: 8-12 mg SQ
  - Can also administer naloxone 2 mg PO: use IV formulation but administer PO

Disposition

- Period of observation depends on agent, onset of action, and duration of effects
  - Heroin: brief observation
  - Methadone, diphenoxylate/atropine: prolonged observation
- Admit
  - Severe, persistent, or worsening signs and symptoms
  - Naloxone infusion after > 1 dose naloxone required

PEARL. Strongly consider for children/elderly
  - Evening: may not be able to adequately be observed at home in the middle of the night

- Long-acting
  - Methadone exposures should be admitted
  - Buprenorphine exposures in children should be observed 12-24 hrs
- Extended release products
— Body packers: either symptomatic or asymptomatic
— Body stuffers: symptomatic
— Whole fentanyl patch ingestions
— Body stuffers: asymptomatic
  - Disposition of asymptomatic body stuffers is controversial
  - Would observe for at least 6 hrs but can consider admission

Loperamide

Source: OTC anti-diarrheal medications
- Increasing use as an abuse agent or opioid substitute
- Increasing use as a mechanism to assist with opioid withdrawal symptoms

Toxic Dose
- Single ingestion < 0.4 mg/kg in patients > 1 year old are unlikely to cause harm
- Safe when used as directed (2-8 mg daily)

PEARL. Larger doses (50-300 mg) can produce CNS and cardiovascular toxicity

Mechanism of Action
- Synthetic phenylpiperidine derivative
- Acts on μ-opioid receptors in the GI tract
- Opioid-like toxicity in overdoses
- If taken with another medication that inhibits P-glycoprotein then concentration can be increased and toxicity can occur

Clinical Manifestations
- Opioid Toxidrome (See Opioids, p. 181)
  — CNS depression
  — Respiratory depression
  — Miosis
- CV
  — Syncope

PEARL. Syncope results from cardiac conduction abnormalities and dysrhythmias

- QT prolongation: torsades de pointes
            - QRS prolongation
    - GI
        - Constipation
        - Ileus
        - Nausea
        - Abdominal cramping

Diagnostics
- Serum concentrations not readily available
- EKG
- BMP

Treatment
- ABCDE
- Respiratory depression: naloxone
    - Adult: Start at 0.04-0.4 mg IV/IM/SQ/IN/IO
        - Repeat dose if initial response not adequate, up to 10 mg total
        - Goal: Titrate to RR ≥ 12 and sufficient tidal volume. If opioid naive, can start with 0.04 mg
    - Pediatric
        - Opioid naïve: 0.01 mg/kg IV (IM, SQ, IO; intratracheal can be used but not preferred)
        - Opioid dependent: 0.001 mg/kg
        - Titrate to effect
    - For recurrent respiratory depression consider infusion
        - Infusion rate: 2/3 of total reversal dose/hr
- QRS prolongation
    - Sodium bicarbonate
        - Bolus: 1-2 mEq/kg IV push over 1-2 min—repeat as necessary q3-5 min to shorten QRS interval
        - Infusion: 150 mEq in 1 L D5W @ 150-200 mL/h (2x maintenance in pediatrics)

        PEARL. Target serum pH 7.55, [Na⁺] 150 mEq/L

    - Lidocaine can be considered for dysrhythmias or persistent cardiotoxicity despite sodium bicarbonate treatment
        - Adult: 1-1.5 mg/kg IV push × 1 over 2 min; repeat 0.5-0.75 mg/kg bolus q5-10min (max cumulative dose: 3 mg/kg). Follow by infusion = 1-4 mg/min; titrate by 1-2 mg/min q10min
            - Infusion rate 20-50 mcg/kg/min

- Pediatric: 1 mg/kg/dose; follow with continuous IV infusion 20-50 mcg/kg/min. May administer second bolus if delay between initial bolus and start of infusion is > 15 min
- QT prolongation: Supplement calcium, potassium, and magnesium as needed
- Torsades de pointes
  - Magnesium
    - 2-4 g SLOW IV at 1 g/min
  - Isoproterenol
    - Initiate @ 5 mcg/min. Titrate by 1 mcg/min q5min to goal BP/HR
    - Usual dose 2-10 mcg/min
  - Overdrive pacing

Disposition

- Admit
  - Severe, persistent, or worsening signs and symptoms or those requiring antidotal treatment
  - Any EKG abnormalities
  - All intentional or large exposures because of delayed and prolonged dysrhythmias

Tramadol

Source

- Pain medications

Toxic Dose

- Can be seen with therapeutic dosing but adverse effects are likely dose dependent

Mechanism of Action

- μ-receptor agonist
- Serotonin reuptake inhibitor
- Tramadol is a prodrug that requires metabolism by CYP2D6 to an active metabolite for its main analgesic effect
  - Ultra-rapid metabolizers can suffer opioid toxicity; has led to fatalities in children
  - Poor metabolizers may receive inadequate analgesia
- Metabolized to inactive metabolites by CYP3A4. CYP3A4 inducers diminish analgesic effects

Clinical Manifestations
- CNS depression
- Respiratory depression

PEARL. Increases risk of seizure even at therapeutic dosing

PEARL. Serotonin syndrome even with therapeutic dosing, more common if combined with other serotonergic agents (See p. 247)

Diagnostics
- Quantitative concentration not available
- Not detected by standard urine drug screens
  - May cause false positive PCP
- Evaluate for complications
  - Head CT: seizures
  - CXR for suspected aspiration, non-cardiogenic pulmonary edema
  - CPK
  - BMP

Treatment
- ABCDE
- Respiratory depression
  - Naloxone
    - Adult: Start at 0.04-0.4 mg IV/IM/IN/IO; repeat dose if initial response not adequate, up to 10 mg total. Titrate to adequate respiratory status. If opioid naive, can start with larger dose, as less concern for precipitating withdrawal
    - Pediatric: Start at 0.04-0.4 mg IV/IM/IN/IO. Repeat dose if initial response not adequate
    - For recurrent respiratory depression consider naloxone infusion: 2/3 of reversal dose infused hourly
    - If not responding to naloxone, airway protection, intubation and mechanical ventilation remains the definitive treatment
- Seizures
  - Diazepam
    - Adult: 5-10 mg IV q5-10min PRN
    - Pediatric: 0.15-0.2 mg/kg IV q5-10min
  - Lorazepam
    - Adult: 2-4 mg IV q5-10min PRN
    - Pediatric: 0.1 mg/kg IV q5-10min PRN
  - Phenobarbital
    - 130-260 mg IV q 20min titrate to effect (in adults)
    - 10 mg/kg IVPB likely to require secure airway

- Propofol (if intubated)
  - Continuous infusion of 5 mcg/kg/min titrate to effect (rec. max of 55 mcg/kg/min)
- Serotonin syndrome (See p. 247)

Disposition
- Observe minimum 6 hrs
- Admit
  - Severe, persistent, or worsening signs and symptoms
  - Requiring > 1 dose naloxone or infusion
  - Intentional extended release ingestions

SALICYLATES

Sources
- Numerous OTC products contain salicylates
- Aspirin (acetylsalicylic acid)
- Oil of wintergreen (methyl salicylate)
- Topical ointments (salicylic acid)
- Bismuth subsalicylate

Toxic Dose
- Acute
  - Mild: 150-200 mg/kg
  - Severe: 300-500 mg/kg
  - Infants and children < 6 years: Lick or taste of oil of wintergreen
  - Children > 6 years: > 4 mL of oil of wintergreen
- Chronic
  - 100 mg/kg/day for > 2 days

Mechanism of Action
- Direct central stimulation of the respiratory center
- Uncoupling of oxidative phosphorylation
- Inhibition of Krebs cycle and fatty acid metabolism
- Alterations in platelet function

Clinical Manifestations
- Acute
  - Tachypnea, hyperpnea
  - N/V
  - Tinnitus/decreased auditory acuity

- Diaphoresis
    - Hyperthermia
    - Altered mental status (consider lower glucose level in CSF than in serum as cause)
    - Hypoglycemia
    - Pulmonary edema
    - Hyperthermia
- Chronic
    - Fewer GI symptoms
    - Tachypnea
    - Tinnitus/decreased auditory acuity
    - Altered mental status
    - Cerebral edema
    - Pulmonary edema
    - Coagulopathy
    - Often older populations

    PEARL. Higher mortality because of delay in diagnosis

Diagnostics

Serum concentration

PEARL. Do NOT wait to obtain salicylate concentration and NEVER use Done nomogram)

- Acute
    - > 30 mg/dL: tinnitus
    - > 90-100 mg/dL: significant toxicity
- Chronic
    - 40-60 mg/dL: significant toxicity
- Repeat salicylate concentrations, BMP, VBG q2hrs until down-trending
- Concentration and toxicity is measured in mg/dL

    PEARL. Careful of units (mg/dL vs. mg/L)

- Specific acid-base dysfunction
    - Early: respiratory alkalosis
    - Late: metabolic acidosis
- BMP
- VBG/ABG
- CXR: Pulmonary edema

Treatment
- ABCDE

  PEARL. Avoid sedation if possible because of blunting of compensatory respiratory response, which can worsen acidosis and result in clinical decompensation

  PEARL. If intubation is required give 2 mEq/kg IV bolus of sodium bicarbonate and hyperventilate prior to sedation/paralysis
  - After intubation MUST attempt to maintain hyperventilation
- Plasma and urinary alkalinization to increase salicylate elimination
  - IV sodium bicarbonate
    - Bolus: 1-2 mEq/kg IVP over 1-2 min
    - Infusion: 150 mEq (3amps) in 1 L D5W with 50 mEQ KCl @ 150-200 mL/h (2x maintenance in pediatrics)
    - Goal serum pH 7.45-7.55
    - Goal urine pH 8.0

    PEARL. Do not mix bicarb in NS or 1/2 NS
- Activated charcoal
  - May be considered if rising salicylate concentration, normal mental status, and tolerating PO or intubated patients via NG/OG
- IVF resuscitation
- Glucose supplementation
- Correct/replete K⁺ to high normal concentration

  PEARL. Aggressive potassium supplementation is needed to successfully alkalinize the urine
- HD
  - Altered mental status
  - Worsening acid-base dysfunction despite aggressive treatment
  - Renal failure
  - Acute: serum concentration > 90 mg/dL
  - Chronic ingestion serum concentration > 60 mg/dL
  - Pulmonary edema

  PEARL. Do not have to wait until concentrations are 90-100 mg/dL acute or 60 mg/dL chronic to dialyze if patient is critically ill and worsening; consult nephrology early

Disposition
- Continue treatment until salicylate concentration < 30 mg/dL
- Discharge when no signs of toxicity and salicylate concentration is down-trending with two levels < 30 mg/dL

- Admit severe, persistent, or worsening signs and symptoms or increasing concentrations despite therapy

PEARL. If signs and symptoms return after treatment cessation because of bezoar formation, a salicylate concentration must be obtained and treatment may need to be restarted.

SEDATIVE/HYPNOTICS

Barbiturates

Source
- Antiepileptic medications
- Migraine medications
- Veterinary euthanasia agents
- Categorized by **onset** and **duration of action**:
  - Ultra-short acting (highly lipid soluble, used for anesthesia)
    - Methohexital
    - Thiopental
  - Short-acting
    - Pentobarbital
    - Secobarbital
  - Intermediate-acting
    - Amobarbital
    - Aprobarbital
    - Butabarbital
    - Butalbital
  - Long-acting
    - Phenobarbital
    - Primidone (2-deoxy-phenobarbital)
    - Mephobarbital

Toxic Dose
- Pentobarbitol: potentially fatal at 2-3 g PO
- Phenobarbitol: potentially fatal at 6-10 g PO

Mechanism of Action
- $GABA_A$ agonist
  - Increases $GABA_A$ activity secondary to increasing the duration of the opening of the Cl- channel
- At high doses, depression of central sympathetic tone

Clinical Manifestations
- Mild toxicity
    - Drowsiness
    - Lethargy
    - Slurred speech
    - Ataxia
    - CNS depression
    - Nystagmus
- Moderate/severe toxicity
    - Hypotension
    - Respiratory depression
    - Coma
    - Hypothermia commonly in comatose patients
    - Barb Blisters—bullous eruptions on pressure points secondary to being down in same position for prolonged period of time
    - Anticipated complications of coma and respiratory depression
        - Aspiration pneumonia/pneumonitis
        - Anoxic brain injury
        - Compartment syndrome/ neuropraxia
- Withdrawal (See Sedative/Hypnotic Withdrawal, p. 265)

Diagnostics
- Toxic Concentration
    - Varies based on drug, route and patient tolerance
- Phenobarbital concentration
    - \> 60 mg/L: Coma
    - \> 80 mg/L: Respiratory depression
    - \> 150-200 mg/L: Hypotension
        - Suspected primidone and phenobarbital toxicity

Treatment
- ABCDE
- Hypotension—IVF resuscitation
- Urinary alkalinization—phenobarbital
- HD for severe ingestions with:
    - Refractory hypotension, renal or cardiac failure
    - Phenobarbital concentration > 100 mcg/mL

Disposition
- Observe minimum 6 hrs
- Admit severe, persistent, or worsening signs and symptoms

Benzodiazepines

Source
- Sedative hypnotic medication

Toxic Dose
- Therapeutic index very high
- Rapid IV injection may cause respiratory depression
- Ingestion of other CNS depressants can produce additive effects

Mechanism of Action
- $GABA_A$ agonist
  - Enhances inhibitory effect of $GABA_A$ by increasing frequency of chloride channel opening

Clinical Manifestations
- Mild toxicity
  - Lethargy
  - Slurred speech
  - Ataxia
  - Hyporeflexia
  - Mid-position pupils
- Severe toxicity (uncommon from oral ingestion more likely with intravenous administration)
  - Coma
  - Hypothermia
  - Respiratory arrest

PEARL. Low risk respiratory depression if oral overdose of a single agent; however high risk in combination with other sedative/hypnotics or opioids

PEARL. Various benzodiazepines have propylene glycol as a diluent and prolonged infusions can cause hyperosmolar lactic acidosis.

- Withdrawal (See Opioid Withdrawal, p. 264)

Diagnostics
- No specific test exists
- Urine drug screening only detects benzodiazepines that are metabolized to oxazepam (diazepam, chlordiazepoxide, temazepam)

Treatment
- ABCDE
- Supportive care and airway protection is typically sufficient
- FluMazenil
  - Use limited due to potential precipitation of withdrawal seizures that are unresponsive to benzodiazepines
  - Contraindications:
    - History of seizures, current seizure activity, cardiac dysrhythmias, co-ingestion of a Na⁺ channel blocking agent or chronic use of benzodiazepines
  - Competitive benzodiazepine receptor antagonist
  - Starting dose: 0.1-0.2 mg IV given over 1 min, repeated as needed in 1 min intervals, to max of 3 mg
  - Pediatric: 0.01 mg/kg (0.2 mg max)
  - Short duration of action (1-2 hrs) leads to re-sedation in up to 65% of patients

PEARL. Indications include: Pediatric ingestion; Reversal of conscious sedation/iatrogenic toxicity; Isolated benzodiazepine overdose in non-tolerant, or not chronically exposed patient

Disposition
- Observe minimum 6 hrs
- Admit severe, persistent, or worsening signs and symptoms or those requiring antidotal treatment

Carisoprodol

Source
- Oral skeletal muscle relaxants

Toxic Dose
- Coma reported after ingestion of 700 mg in 2-year-old
- Death reported after ingestion of 3500 mg in 4-year-old

Mechanism of Action
- CNS depression via $GABA_A$ agonism by meprobamate the metabolite of carisoprodol

PEARL. Meprobamate can produce euphoria, its abuse potential is well-established

- Meprobamate can directly open the $GABA_A$ Cl- channel

Clinical Manifestations
- Lethargy
- Slurred speech
- Ataxia
- Respiratory depression
- Hypotension from direct myocardial depression

PEARL. In overdose spastic encephalopathy, hyperreflexia, opisthotonus, increased muscle tone and myoclonus (including ocular) are common

Diagnostics
- No specific test exists

Treatment
- ABCDE
- Supportive care: Airway protection

Disposition
- Observe minimum 6 hrs
- Admit severe, persistent, or worsening signs and symptoms

Baclofen

Sources
- Intrathecal pump solution
- Oral tablet or liquid formulation

Toxic Dose
- Adults: 200 mg ingestion
- Infants/children: 120 mg ingestion
- Intrathecal: 1.5 mg

Mechanism of Action
- $GABA_B$ agonist

Clinical Manifestations
- **Toxicity**—CNS depression, bradycardia, hypotension, hypotonia, hypothermia and seizure
- **Withdrawal**—Encephalopathy, tachycardia, hypertension, fever, seizure, tremor, and increased spasticity/muscle tone

PEARL. Toxicity in those with renal dysfunction; can develop delirium, agitation, and dystonia

PEARL. Seizures occur in toxicity and in withdrawal

PEARL. Baclofen toxicity can mimic brain death

Diagnostics
- Serum concentrations not readily available
- Intrathecal pump interrogation
- BMP

Treatment
- ABCDE
- HD

   PEARL. Multiple case studies show increased clearance with dialysis in those with decreased renal function

- Intrathecal
  — Interrogation of pump to determine excess or lack of medication delivered
  — Intrathecal washout to decrease CSF concentration of baclofen
- Withdrawal
  — Restart baclofen via the same route if possible
  — Treat with GABA agonist
  — Diazepam
    - Adult: 5-10 mg IV q5-10min PRN
    - Pediatric: 0.2-0.5 mg/kg IV q5-10min
  — Lorazepam
    - Adult: 2-4 mg IV q10-15min PRN
    - Pediatric: 0.05-0.1 mg/kg IV q10-15min PRN
  — Phenobarbital
    - 130-260 mg IV q20min titrate to effect (in adults)
    - 10 mg/kg IVPB may require secure airway
  — Propofol (if intubated)
    - Continuous infusion of 5 mcg/kg/min titrate (rec. max of 55 mcg/kg/min)

Disposition
- Admit severe, persistent, or worsening signs and symptoms or withdrawal

Gamma-hydroxybutyrate (GHB)

Source
- Endogenous neuromodulator related to GABA
- Sodium oxybate, prescribed for narcolepsy
- Drug of abuse

Toxic Dose
- \> 20-30 mg/kg results in CNS depression
- \> 50-70 mg/kg results in coma, respiratory depression

Mechanism of Action
- $GABA_B$ agonist, GHB receptor agonist

Clinical Manifestation
- CNS depression
- Respiratory depression
- Myoclonus
- Bradycardia

PEARL. Rapid onset CNS/respiratory depression with improvement in several hours

PEARL. Drug of abuse in bodybuilders, date-rape drug; chronic use can lead to tolerance and dependence

Diagnostics
- Quantitative concentration only available from reference lab

Treatment
- ABCDE
- Ensure adequate airway protection, oxygenation and ventilation
- Social work to facilitate police report for suspected drug facilitated assault
- Determine if sexual assault forensic exam is indicated

Disposition
- Toxicity will often resolve within several hours of an acute ingestion
- Admit severe, persistent, or worsening signs and symptoms

"Z-Drugs" Imidazopyridine Hypnotic

Sources
- Zolpidem
- Zopiclone
- Zaleplon

Toxic Dose
- Toxic/therapeutic ratio generally high but can product additive effects when combined with other sedative hypnotics

Mechanism of Action
- Selectively binds to α-1 subunits of $GABA_A$ receptor and acts as an agonist, enhancing chloride ion influx and cellular hyperpolarization

PEARL. Structurally unrelated to benzodiazepines but exhibit similar adverse drug effects, toxicity, and even withdrawal although mild in comparison

Clinical Manifestations
- CNS depression typically without significant respiratory depression

  PEARL. Parasomnia may precipitate accidents
  - Ataxia
  - Slurred speech

Diagnostics
- Quantitative concentration not available
- Do not cross react with benzodiazepine immunoassay

Treatment
- ABCDE

Disposition
- Observe minimum 6 hrs
- Admit severe, persistent, or worsening signs and symptoms

PESTICIDES/RODENTICIDES

PESTICIDES

Aluminum Phosphide

Sources
- Agricultural fumigant
- Rodenticide
- Possible byproduct of home methamphetamine labs

Toxic Dose

PEARL. Phosphine gas upon contact with water
- Inhaled or absorbed through respiratory and GI tract
  - 1-3 ppm
    PEARL. Detectable "fishy" odor
  - 50 ppm IDLH
- Phosphide: Ingested
  - Forms phosphine gas on contact with water, which is enhanced in acidic environment
  - As little as 500 mg can be fatal

Mechanism of Action
- Disrupts oxidative phosphorylation by inhibiting cytochrome c oxidase
- Generates radial oxygen species

Clinical Manifestations
- GI
  - Profuse vomiting and abdominal pain are usually first symptoms if tablets are ingested

  PEARL. As phosphide reacts with gastric acid, phosphine gas is produced and absorbed by both respiratory and GI tracts
  - Elevated LFT
- CNS
  - Depression
  - Coma
  - Seizure

- CV
  - Shock
  - Dysrhythmias
- Pulmonary
  - Acute lung injury
  - ARDS

Diagnostics
- EKG
- CMP
- ABG
- CXR in those with respiratory symptoms

Treatment
- ABCDE/Supportive care: Most important first step
  - Early airway intervention for respiratory distress or coma
- Universal precautions should be employed
- Consider gastric lavage if ingested
- Although not routinely used in poisonings given the severity of phosphine toxicity it can be considered in patients who present early in the course (< 1 hr)

  PEARL. Gastric contents may result in gas phosphine; use caution

- Seizures
  - Diazepam
    - Adult: 5-10 mg IV q5-10min PRN
    - Pediatric: 0.2-0.5 mg/kg IV q5-10min
  - Lorazepam
    - Adult: 2-4 mg IV q15min PRN
    - Pediatric: 0.05-0.1 mg/kg IV q15min PRN
  - Phenobarbital
    - 130-260 mg IV q 20min titrate to effect (in adults)
    - 10 mg/kg IVPB likely to require secure airway
  - Propofol (if intubated)
    - Continuous infusion of 5 mcg/kg/min titrate (rec. max of 55 mcg/kg/min)
- Hypotension
  - IVF
  - Titrate direct acting vasopressors, such as norepinephrine

- Metabolic acidosis
  - Sodium bicarbonate
    - Bolus: 1-2 mEq/kg IVP over 1-2 min
    - Infusion: 100-150 mEq in 1 L D5W @ 150-200 mL/h (2x maintenance in pediatrics)
- ECMO for refractory shock

Disposition
- Admit all

Organophosphates & Carbamates

Sources
- Insecticides
- Pesticides
- Chemical weapons

Toxic Dose
- Varies greatly
- Exposure can be through ingestion, inhalation, or dermal routes

Mechanism of Action
- Acetylcholinesterase (AchE) inhibitor—blocks the breakdown of acetylcholine
- Increases synaptic acetylcholine (Ach) concentrations
- Can have muscarinic, nicotinic, or both receptors stimulated
- If not reversed in time, "aging" process will occur
  - Aging: the inhibited AchE will no longer be able to regenerate and will have to wait for the body to produce more AchE
  - Carbamates do not undergo "aging"

Clinical Manifestations
- Occur in 3 general categories
  - Muscarinic
  - Nicotinic
  - CNS

- Muscarinic effects
  - **SLUDGE or DUMBELS**
    - **S**alivation
    - **L**acrimation
    - **U**rination
    - **D**efecation
    - **G**I distress
    - **E**mesis
    - **D**iarrhea
    - **U**rination
    - **M**iosis
    - **B**ronchorrhea
    - **E**xcessive **L**acrimation
    - **S**alivation
  - **Killer B's: B**ronchorrhea, **B**ronchospasm, **B**radycardia
- Nicotinic effects
  - Hypertension
  - Tachycardia
  - Bronchodilator
  - Muscle cramping and fasciculations
  - Mydriasis
- CNS effects
  - Restlessness
  - Confusion
  - Ataxia
  - Tremors
  - Seizure
  - Coma

Diagnostics
- RBC cholinesterase
  - Correlates with CNS toxicity at the NMJ
  - Regenerates at 1% per day
  - Wide interpersonal variability in baseline concentration and amount needed to be lost to have clinical symptoms
  - False depression
    - Pernicious anemia
    - Hemoglobinopathies
  - No readily available laboratory test

- Plasma/butyrylcholinesterase
  - Less specific than RBC cholinesterase
  - False depression
    - Liver disease
    - Malnutrition
    - Pregnancy
  - Declines faster and normalizes faster than RBC cholinesterase
  - Metabolizes other agents
    - Cocaine
    - Succinylcholine
    - Pyrethroid insecticides
- Electromyogram (EMG)
  - Used in rebound cholinergic presentations or Intermediate Syndrome

Treatment
- ABCDE
- Decontamination
  - PPE such as neoprene gloves and gown
  - Remove and dispose of all patient clothing as hazardous waste
  - Thoroughly cleanse patient with soap and water
  - If ophthalmologic exposure is suspected, irrigate eyes

PEARL. Avoid succinylcholine as a paralytic secondary to prolonged effects of the medication because it is metabolized by plasma acetylcholinesterase

- Atropine
  - Treats muscarinic symptoms
  - Escalating doses: 2-5 mg every 5 min
  - Administer until muscarinic symptoms are controlled
    - Endpoint: control of bronchorrhea and bronchospasm, no more vomiting or diarrhea, dry skin and mucosa, then start infusion
  - Infusion rate: 10-20% of total loading atropine dose that was needed to obtain control
  - Tachycardia is not contraindication
- Pralidoxime
  - Regenerates AchE by displacing organophosphate from AchE prior to aging
  - Dosing regimens vary
    - 1-2 g IV over 10 min followed by infusion 500 mg/hr IV
    - 1-2 g IV over 10 min, then 1- 2 g q6hrs for 48-72 hrs
    - Effectiveness is currently still debated

- Has no effect on aged acetylcholinesterase
  - Aging takes from 6 min-72 hrs depending on the agent

PEARL. Pralidoxime is not indicated for carbamate exposures since no aging occurs

Disposition
- Admit all symptomatic patients

RODENTICIDES

Barium

Sources
- Most common clinically significant exposures
  - Ingestion
    - Rodenticides
    - Insecticides
    - Depilatories (hair removal products)
  - Fireworks ("color snakes" and "black snakes")
- Soluble barium salts such as barium carbonate, chloride, nitrate

PEARL. GI contrast agent barium sulfate ($BaSO_4$) is insoluble and non-toxic

Toxic Dose
- Ingestions of 0.2 g of barium salts may be toxic
- Lethal doses in humans usually range 1-30 g

Mechanism of Action
- K^+ efflux channel blockade leading to intracellular sequestration of potassium

Clinical Manifestations

PEARL. Toxicity associated with paresthesia around the mouth and neck

- 45-90 min post ingestion
  - Earliest symptoms
    - N/V/D
    - Abdominal pain
- 2-3 hrs post ingestion

PEARL. Paresthesia of hands and feet with severe hypokalemia

- > 3 hrs
  - CNS effects
    - Flaccid muscle weakness
    - Hyporeflexia
    - Flaccid paralysis
  - Respiratory failure because of muscle weakness
  - Ventricular dysrhythmias because of hypokalemia
  - Lactic acidosis and rhabdomyolysis

Diagnostics
- EKG
- Serial BMP
- Mg^{2+}
- PO_4^-
- Ca^{2+}
- Lactate

Treatment
- ABCDE
- Consider gastric lavage
- Oral magnesium sulfate to prevent further barium absorption
  - Adult: 30 g
  - Pediatric: 250 mg/kg
- Potassium supplementation
- HD
  - Consider for severe poisoning with refractory hypokalemia and/or muscle weakness

Disposition
- Observe minimum 6 hrs
- Admit severe, persistent, or worsening signs and symptoms

Sodium Monofluoroacetate and Fluoroacetamide

Source
- "Toxic sheep collars" (coyotes who kill sheep likely to puncture collar and become poisoned)

Toxic Dose
- Estimated 2-10 mg/kg may be lethal in humans

Mechanism of Action
- Must be absorbed metabolized to fluorocitrate, an Irreversible inhibitor of the TCA (Krebs) cycle

Clinical Manifestations
- Often within 1 hr of ingestion, but may be delayed up to 20 hrs
  - N/V/D
  - Abdominal pain
- Initial symptoms followed by
  - Diaphoresis
  - Altered mental status/agitation
  - Seizure
  - Coma
  - Metabolic acidosis
  - Hypocalcemia
  - Respiratory arrest
  - Cardiovascular collapse

Diagnostics
- BMP

  PEARL. Hypo/hyperglycemia and hypocalcemia
- CBC
- Lactate
- NH_3
- ABG
- EKG

Treatment
- ABCDE: Maximize supportive care and early intubation for severe toxicity
- IVF followed by vasopressors for hypotension
- Benzodiazepines for agitation and seizure activity
- Monitor for dysrhythmias
- Consider gastric lavage and activated charcoal if < 1 hr
- Glycerol monoacetate and sterile IV ethanol are unproven therapies
- Electrolyte correction (hypocalcemia)

Disposition
- Admit all symptomatic patients

Strychnine

Sources
- Pest control agent (moles, gophers, pigeons)
- *Strychnos Nux*-vomica

Toxic Dose
- Adult: 10-20 mg (deaths reported at 5 mg)
- Pediatric: 2 mg

Mechanism of Action
- Competitive antagonist of the inhibitory neurotransmitter glycine at the ventral horn motor neurons in the spinal cord
- Increased motor neuronal excitability leading to increased muscular activity

Clinical Manifestations

PEARL. Watch for respiratory compromise because of respiratory muscle spasms

- 10-30 min after ingestion
  - Heightened awareness
  - AMS
  - Severe cramps
  - Hyperreflexia
  - Hyperthermia
  - Tachycardia
  - Rhabdomyolysis
  - Metabolic acidosis
  - Renal failure
  - Risus sardonicus
  - Opisthotonus

PEARL. Excess motor activity- painful diffuse muscle contractions that resembles convulsions however consciousness is maintained

Diagnostics
- BMP
- CPK
- Lactate

Treatment
- ABCDE

> **PEARL.** Treatment focuses on cessation of excess motor activity and airway control. Early sedation, neuromuscular paralysis, and airway control can prevent death in severe cases.

- Avoid stimulation as this can precipitate muscle spasms
- Excess Motor Activity
  - Diazepam
    - Adult: 5-10 mg IV q5-10min PRN
    - Pediatric: 0.2-0.5 mg/kg IV q5-10min
  - Lorazepam
    - Adult: 2-4 mg IV q15min PRN
    - Pediatric: 0.05-0.1 mg/kg IV q15min PRN
  - Phenobarbital
    - 130-260 mg IV q 20min titrate to effect (in adults)
    - 10 mg/kg IVPB likely to require secure airway
  - Propofol (if intubated)
    - Continuous infusion of 5 mcg/kg/min titrate (rec. max of 55 mcg/kg/min)
- Resistant Excess Motor Activity
  - NON-depolarizing neuromuscular blockers (paralysis)
  - Succinylcholine relatively contraindicated
- Rhabdomyolysis
  - IVF to ensure adequate urine output; goal 2-3 mL/kg/hr
  - Alkalinization can be considered
  - Monitor renal function

Disposition
- Observe 12 hrs: unintentional asymptomatic patients
- Admit all symptomatic patients

Superwarfarins

Sources
- Residential and industrial grade rodent control agents
- 4-OH-coumarins
  - Brodifacoum
  - Bromadiolone
  - Difenacoum

- Indanedione
    - Chlorophacinone
    - Diphacinone
    - Pindone
- Most common rodenticide exposures in the U.S. are 4-OH-coumarins (> 90% of exposures)
- Most are unintentional ingestions in age < 6 years old
- Most serious toxicity is from intentional ingestion

Toxic Dose
- Children
    - > 25 g 0.005% 4-OH-coumarin

Mechanism of Action
- Competitive inhibition of vitamin K epoxide reductase leading to deficit of Vit-K dependent factors (II, VII, IX, X)

Clinical Manifestations

PEARL. Earliest sign of coagulopathy is often hematuria

- Bleeding can occur at any site
    - Epistaxis
    - Hemarthrosis
    - Dysmenorrhea
    - Hematuria
    - Intracranial bleeding
    - Intraabdominal or retroperitoneal bleeding
- Coagulopathy lasting up to 9 months possible (half-life 16-34 days)
- Patients likely asymptomatic up to 72 hrs after ingestion

Diagnostics

PEARL. No diagnostics are necessary in asymptomatic child who ingested < 25 g or who presents < 24 hrs after ingestion

- LFT
- PT/INR (serial measurements)
- CBC
- Type and screen/cross for life-threatening hemorrhage
- Quantitative superwarfarin concentrations can be performed by reference laboratories
    - May be necessary in patients who deny ingestion/self-poisoning or suspected Munchausen syndrome by proxy

Treatment

- Most unintentional ingestions will not need treatment
- ABCDE
- See algorithm
- Consider activated charcoal
- Active hemorrhage
  - Fluid resuscitation and transfusion of blood products in accordance with degree of hemorrhage
  - Administer 4-Factor PCC
    - Re-dose if hemorrhage uncontrolled
  - Vitamin K1/phytonadione
    - Adult: 10 mg IV
    - Pediatric: 1-5 mg IV
    - Re-dose q6hrs if persistently elevated INR
    - High doses may be required

    PEARL. Patient may need long duration of treatment after active hemorrhage controlled

    - Adult: 25-50 mg PO TID-QID × 1-2 days, then per INR
    - Pediatric: 5-10 mg (0.4 mg/kg/dose) BID-QID × 1-2 days, then per INR
    - FFP
      - Associated with standard risks of blood product transfusion
      - Volume required may prevent its use in patients with renal failure or congestive heart failure
      - Titrate to prothrombin
      - May have to readminister after 4-6 hrs

Disposition

- See Algorithm

Management Algorithm

Superwarfarin ingestion known or suspected

Asymptomatic

- < 25 g of 0.005% 4-OH-coumarin
- \> 25 g of 0.005% 4-OH-coumarin
  - < 24 hrs since ingestion
    - GI decontamination with activated charcoal if with 1 hr of ingestion
    - No routine PT/INR or Vitamin K needed
    - May be discharged with instructions to monitor for signs of bleeding and have a PT drawn 24 & 48 hrs from ingestion. If intentional ingestion, then admit to psychiatry and follow PT/INR as described
      - Normal PT/INR at 24 & 48 hrs— no further work-up needed
      - Prolonged PT/INR: Vitamin K1, monitor for bleeding, F/U in 24 hrs
  - \> 24 hrs since ingestion

Discharge; no F/U labs needed; psychiatry eval if intentional

Symptomatic: signs of coagulopathy and bleeding

- Oxygen, IV fluids, consider 4 factor PCC, FFP for active bleeding, Vit K (10 mg adults, 1-5 mg in children), transfuse if needed
- Laboratory tests: PT/INR, CBC, CMP, Type and crossmatch
- Admit; ICU vs floor depends on degree of bleeding and coagulopathy; psychiatry eval if intentional
- Check PT/INR
  - Abnormal: Vitamin K1, F/U in 24 hrs
  - Normal: F/U PT/INR at 48 hrs. If normal, nothing further

Psychiatry eval and consider admit if intentional

PLANTS

ACKEE FRUIT (*BLIGHIA SAPIDA*)

Sources
- Fruit of the ackee tree, edible when ripe but toxic in all other states

Mechanism of Action
- Hypoglycin A/B: metabolized to toxic metabolite methylene cyclopropyl acetic acid (MCPA), which combines with coenzyme A; MCPA-CoA is a suicide inhibitor
- Inhibition of acyl-CoA dehydrogenase prevents the β-oxidation of fatty acids
- Mitochondrial toxicity

Clinical Manifestations
PEARL. "Jamaican vomiting sickness"
- GI
  - N/V
  - Steatosis
  - Hepatic failure
- Metabolic
  - Hypoglycemia
  - Metabolic acidosis
  - Hyperammonemia
- CNS
  - Seizures

Diagnostics
- BMP
- LFT
- NH_3

Treatment
- ABCDE
- Hypoglycemia: IV or oral dextrose
  - Oral glucose gel or tablets available while securing IV access
  - D5W or D10W infusion titrated to maintain euglycemia
    - 0.5-1.0 g/kg, adjust based on size

- If concentration > D12.5W central venous access needed
  - Adult: D50 (0.5 g/mL) IV
  - Pediatric: D25 (0.25 g/mL) IV
  - Neonates: D10 (0.1 g/mL) IV
- Consider administering thiamine if deficient
■ Metabolic acidosis/liver failure
- L-carnitine (although unproven, may be beneficial)
  - Loading dose: 100 mg/kg IV (max 6 g) over 15-30 min, then 15 mg/kg (max 3 g per dose) IV q4hrs over 10-30 min
  - Prophylaxis: 100 mg/kg/d PO divided q6hrs (max 3 g/day in adults and 2 g/day in children)

Disposition
■ Admit severe, persistent, or worsening signs and symptoms or those requiring antidotal treatment

ANTIMUSCARINIC PLANTS

Sources
■ *Atropa bella-donna*
■ *Mandragora officinarum*
■ *Datura stramonium*
■ *Hyoscyamus niger*
■ *Brugmansia* sp.

Mechanism of Action
■ Contains scopolamine, hyoscyamine, a component of atropine, and other tropane alkaloids that cause an anti-cholinergic effect

Clinical Manifestations
■ Antimuscarinic (See Antihistamines & Antimuscarinics, p. 151)

Diagnostics
■ No specific test

Treatment
■ ABCDE
■ Antimuscarinic delirium (See Antihistamines & Antimuscarinics, p. 151)

Disposition
■ Admit severe, persistent, or worsening signs and symptoms or those requiring antidotal treatment

CARDIAC GLYCOSIDE PLANTS

Sources
- *Convallaria majalis* (Lily of the Valley)
- *Urginea maritima* (red squill)
- *Thevitia peruviana* (yellow oleander)
- *Nerium oleander* (common oleander)
- *Digitalis purpurea* (foxglove)

Mechanism of Action
- Contains cardiac glycoside, which inhibits Na^+K^- ATPase

Clinical Manifestations
- See Digoxin Chapter, p. 172

Diagnostics
- Serum digoxin concentration
    - **PEARL.** May not reflect degree of toxicity
- EKG
- BMP
    - **PEARL.** Hyperkalemia

Treatment
- ABCDE
- Life-threatening dysrhythmia/hyperkalemia
    — Digoxin immune FAB
        - No specific treatment guidelines
        - Consider 10 vials IV empirically for critically ill patient

Disposition
- Admit severe, persistent, or worsening signs and symptoms or those requiring antidotal treatment

CARDIOTOXIC NA^+ BLOCKERS

Sources
- Yew plant

Mechanism of Action
- Na^+ channel blockade

Clinical Manifestations
- GI
  - N/V
- CV
  - QRS prolongation
  - Tachycardia
  - Bradycardia
- CNS
  - Seizures

Diagnostics
- EKG

Treatment
- ABCDE
- Bradycardia: Atropine
  - Adult: 0.5 mg q3-5min
  - Pediatric: 0.02 mg/kg IV (minimum dose 0.1 mg when > 5 kg, max doses 0.5 mg) q3-5min
- QRS prolongation or hypotension: IV sodium bicarbonate
  - Bolus: 1-2 mEq/kg IVP over 1-2 min
  - Infusion: 100-150 mEq in 1 L D5W @ 150-200 mL/h (2x maintenance in pediatrics)

Disposition
- Admit severe, persistent, or worsening signs and symptoms or those requiring antidotal treatment

CARDIOTOXIC NA$^+$ CHANNEL OPENERS

Sources
- *Rhododendron*
- *Aconitum*
- *Toxicoscordion venenosum*
- *Veratrum viride*
- *Andromeda*

Mechanism of Action
- Cardiac Na$^+$ channel opening

Clinical Manifestations
- GI
  - N/V
- CV
  - Bradycardia
  - Hypotension
  - Dysrhythmias
  - Syncope

PEARL. Presentation is similar to digoxin toxicity, except serum K⁺ is normal

Diagnostics
- EKG
- BMP
- Serum digoxin concentration
- CPK
- Troponin

Treatment
- ABCDE
- Bradycardia: Atropine
  - Adult: 0.5 mg q3-5min
  - Pediatric: 0.02 mg/kg IV (minimum dose 0.1 mg when > 5 kg, max doses 0.5 mg) q3-5min
- Hypotension: Vasopressors for fluid resistant hypotension
- Ventricular arrhythmias: May be resistant to antiarrhythmic agents (can try lidocaine)
- ECMO/cardiopulmonary bypass

Disposition
- Admit severe, persistent, or worsening signs and symptoms

COLCHICINE

Sources
- *Colchicum autumnale* L. (Autumn crocus)
- *Gloriosa superba* (flame lily)

PEARL. Gout medication

Mechanism of Action
- Microtubule inhibitor

Clinical Manifestations
- GI
  - N/V/D
- Heme
  - Initial leukocytosis followed by leukopenia

> **PEARL.** Bone marrow suppression

- CV
  - CV collapse
  - Multisystem organ failure (renal failure, hepatic failure, etc.)
- CNS
  - Neuropathy
- Derm
  - Alopecia

Diagnostics
- BMP
- CBC

Treatment
- ABCDE
- Aggressive supportive care
- HD or CRRT for renal failure
- Bone marrow suppression: consider G-CSF

Disposition
- Admit severe, persistent, or worsening signs and symptoms or those requiring antidotal treatment

HEMLOCK–POISON (*CONIUM MACULATUM*)

Source
- All parts of the plant are toxic
- Often confused with edibles

Mechanism of Action
- Contains coniine, which is structurally similar to nicotine with resulting early stimulation of acetylcholine receptors in the CNS and PNS
- Followed by late paradoxical blocking of acetylcholine receptors

Clinical Manifestations
- Nicotinic signs and symptoms
  - N/V/D, tachycardia, hypertension, diaphoresis, fasciculations
  - Followed by hypotension, muscle weakness, respiratory failure
- Cholinergic Toxidrome (See Toxidrome Table, p. 282)

Diagnostics
- No specific test

Treatment
- ABCDE
- Aggressive supportive care
- IVF, intubation, vasopressors/inotropes

Disposition
- Admit severe, persistent, or worsening signs and symptoms

HEMLOCK—WATER (*CICUTA MACULATA*)

Source
- All parts of the plant are toxic
- Often confused with edibles

Mechanism of Action
- Contains cicutoxin (potent neurotoxin), which acts as an antagonist at the $GABA_A$ receptor

Clinical Manifestations
- N/V/D

PEARL. Seizures within 1-3 hrs
- Seizures may be refractory/status epilepticus
- Shock/cardiovascular collapse

Diagnostics
PEARL. Often confused with edible plants
- No specific test

Treatment
- ABCDE
- Seizures
  - Diazepam
    - Adult: 5-10 mg IV q5 mins PRN
    - Pediatric: 0.2 mg/kg IV q5min
  - Lorazepam
    - Adult: 2-4 mg IV q15min PRN
    - Pediatric: 0.1 mg/kg IV
      - Repeat 0.1 mg/kg q15min
  - Phenobarbital (if benzodiazepines ineffective)
    - 20 mg/kg IVPB
  - Propofol (if intubated)
    - 1-2 mg/kg IV bolus followed by continuous infusion 20 mcg/kg/min

Disposition
- Admit severe, persistent, or worsening signs and symptoms

INSOLUBLE OXALATES

Sources
- Dieffenbachia
- Philodendron
- Elephant's ear

Mechanism of Action
- Ca^{2+} oxalate crystals

Clinical Manifestations

PEARL. Common pediatric exposure when leaves are chewed

- GI
  - Oropharyngeal edema
  - Swelling
  - Dysphagia

Diagnostics
- No specific test

Treatment
- ABCDE
- Ice or cool compresses
- NSAIDS

Disposition
- Admit severe, persistent, or worsening signs and symptoms

NICOTINE

Sources
- *Nicotiana tabacum*
- Blue cohosh
- *Sophora secundiflora*

Mechanism of Action
- Activates Ach receptors in the CNS and PNS

Clinical Manifestations
- Cholinergic toxidrome (See Toxidrome Table, p. 282)

PEARL. Green tobacco sickness in plant handlers because of dermal absorption

Diagnosis
- No specific test

Treatment
- ABCDE

Disposition
- Admit severe, persistent, or worsening signs and symptoms

PHYTOLACCA AMERICANA (POKEWEED)

Sources
- Plants in this species include pokeweed, inkberry, pigeonberry, pokeberry, common pokeweed, phytolaque d'Amerique, poke, American pokeweed

Mechanism of Action
- Pokeweed mitogen

PEARL. Parboiling negates toxicity

Clinical Manifestations
- N/V/D

PEARL. Often purple stained to lips and fingers

Diagnostics
- BMP
- CBC (plasmacytosis)

Treatment
- ABCDE
- Supportive care with IVFs and antiemetics

Disposition
- Admit severe, persistent, or worsening signs and symptoms

TOXALBUMINS

Sources
- *Ricinus communis* (castor bean)
- *Abrus precatorius* (Jequerity bean, rosary pea)

Mechanism of Action
- Inhibits protein synthesis by inactivating the 60S ribosomal subunits

Clinical Manifestations
PEARL. Non-chewed seeds do not cause toxicity
- GI
  — N/V/D
  — Hematochezia
- CV
  — Shock
  — Multi-organ system failure

Diagnostics
- CBC
- BMP
- LFT

Treatment
- ABCDE

Disposition
- Admit severe, persistent, or worsening signs and symptoms

TOXICODENDRON

Sources
- Poison ivy
- Poison sumac
- Poison oak

Mechanism of Action
- Type IV hypersensitivity reaction to urushiol in plant leaf

Clinical Manifestations
- Derm
  - Vesiculo-bullous, linear rash that may ooze, crust, and scale

PEARL. Can re-inoculate with contact with residual resin on clothing or animal fur

Diagnostics
- No specific test

Treatment
- Topical steroids
- Systemic steroids
  - Severe, diffuse
  - Facial involvement
- Antihistamines

Disposition
- Discharge

PEARL. Rebound rash may occur if poison ivy is not treated with an extended course of steroids

SUBSTANCES OF ABUSE

HALLUCINOGENS & OTHER PSYCHOTROPICS

Note: Diagnostics, treatments, and disposition for all psychotropic agents are similar and are listed at end of the chapter.

Dextromethorphan

Sources
- Component of cough/cold medications
- Is an opioid but lacks analgesic properties (optical isomer of levorphanol)

Toxic Dose
- Moderate: > 10 mg/kg
- Severe: > 20-30 mg/kg

Mechanism of Action
- Antagonism of the NMDA receptor
- Inhibits reuptake of serotonin

Clinical Manifestations
- Mild
  - N/V
  - Nystagmus
  - Tachycardia
  - Hypertension
  - Altered mental status
  - Auditory and visual hallucinations
  - Mydriasis or miosis
  - Ataxia
- Severe
  - Stupor
  - Coma
  - Seizures
  - Hyperthermia
  - Respiratory depression
- May cause serotonin syndrome (See Serotonin Syndrome, p. 247)
  - Hyperthermia
  - Muscle rigidity
  - Altered mental status
  - Hypertension

- Often co-formulated with other substances
  - Acetaminophen (See Acetaminophen/Paracetamol, p. 95)
  - Antihistamines (See Antihistamines & Antimuscarinics, p. 151)

Ketamine

Sources
- Available as street drug and for medical/veterinary use

Toxic Dose
- Intranasal: 10-250 mg
- Oral/rectal: 40-450 mg
- IM: 10-100 mg

Mechanism of Action
- Psychotropic effects: Antagonism of the NMDA receptor
- Anesthetic effects: Agonism of the M, Δ, Σ, and K opioid receptors

Clinical Manifestations
- ACUTE (effects are dose-dependent and similar to those seen with ketamine sedation in medical setting)
  - Hallucinations (commonly described as dysphoric)
  - Hypersalivation
  - Lacrimation
  - Nystagmus
  - Hypertension
  - Tachycardia
- Emergence reaction
  - Acute psychosis during the recovery phase: confusion, vivid dreams, hallucinations
- CHRONIC
  - Abdominal and pelvic pain
  - Memory loss

Lysergamides (Natural)

Sources
- Derivatives of lysergic acid
  - Lysergic acid amide—in morning glory seeds
  - Ergine—in Hawaiian baby woodrose
  - Lysergic acid diethylamide (LSD)

Toxic Dose
- Variable; some effects (entactogenic) not dose-dependent while others (sympathomimetic, hallucinations) are

Mechanism of Action
- Serotonin (5HT2) and dopamine agonist mediating release of excitatory neurotransmitters
- 5HT2A receptors are thought to mediate hallucinosis

Clinical Manifestations
- Visual and auditory hallucinations or illusions, synesthesias, body dysmorphisms
- Mild sympathomimetic symptoms including tachycardia

Lysergic Acid Diethylamide (LSD)

Source
- Synthetic chemical derived from research on ergot alkaloids of the fungus, *Claviceps purpurea*

Toxic Dose
- Doses of 1-1.5 mcg/kg produce psychedelic effects, with the dosage for typical LSD reaction estimated to be in the range of 100-200 mcg
  - Tolerance with repeated use and cross-tolerance has been demonstrated between LSD, mescaline, and psilocybin

Mechanism of Action
- 5HT2A and dopamine agonist mediating release of excitatory neurotransmitters

Clinical Manifestations
- Psychedelic effects within 30 min of ingestion, peak within 4 hrs, duration 8-12 hrs
  - Euphoria
  - Visual and auditory hallucinations or illusions, synesthesias, body dysmorphisms
  - Paranoia
  - Impulsivity
- Sympathomimetic stimulation usually precedes the psychedelic effects
  - Mydriasis
  - Tachycardia
  - Hypertension

- In massive overdoses, coagulopathy, hyperthermia, seizure, coma, and respiratory arrest have been reported

PEARL. Chronic use may lead to hallucinogen persisting perception disorder—recurrent perceptual disturbances similar to acute intoxication, and triggered by stress, illness, or other stimulus in the absence of drug

Mescaline

Sources
- Mescaline (3, 4, 5-trimethoxyphenethylamine) found in peyote and other cacti

Toxic Dose
- Typically, 3-12 "buttons" or 200-500 mg
- Onset 30-60 min, duration 5-12 hrs, though wide individual variability
- No known lethal dose

Mechanism of Action
- Thought to be serotonergic agonist, but much less potent than LSD

Clinical Manifestations
- Onset within 1 hr; duration approximately 6-12 hrs
- GI
  - N/V
  - Abdominal discomfort
- CV
  - Diaphoresis
  - Tachycardia
  - Hypertension
  - Hyperthermia
- CNS
  - Mydriasis
  - Nystagmus
  - Ataxia
  - Headache
  - Altered sensorium
  - Altered sense of time
  - Visual, auditory hallucinations and illusions

Nutmeg

Sources
- Dried seed from the tropical *Myristica fragrans* tree

Toxic Dose
- Ingestion of 1-3 nutmegs or 5-15 g of the ground spice produces psychologic effects

Mechanism of Action
- The hallucinogenic properties of nutmeg may be caused by the component myristicin; mechanism is not well understood

Clinical Manifestations
- Hallucinogenic and adrenergic effects typically occur 3-6 hrs after ingestion and can last 6-24 hrs
- GI
  - N/V/D
  - Abdominal pain
- CV
  - Tachycardia
  - Flushing
- CNS
  - Dry Mouth
  - Hallucinations

Salvia

Sources
- Perennial herb in the mint family

Toxic Dose
- Often smoked, chewed, held sublingually or buccally, or ingested in tea
- When smoked:
  - Typically, dose of 200-500 mcg, has < 1 min onset
  - Tapers over 10-20 min
  - May last up to 1-2 hrs

Mechanism of Action
- Salvinorin A is an agonist of kappa opioid receptors

Clinical Manifestations
- Hallucinations
- Diaphoresis
- Diuresis
- Dysphoria
- Uncontrollable laughter
- Altered perception of sensation, particularly synesthesias
- Headache
- Few reports of psychosis and suicide associated with use

Tryptamines (Indolealkylamines)

Sources
- Natural
  - Psilocybin (4-phosphoryloxy-N, N-dimethyltryptamine) and psilocin (4-hydroxy-N, N-dimethyltryptamine): from "magic mushrooms"
  - 5-MeO-DMT (5-methoxy-N, N-dimethyltryptamine): from secretions of *Bufo* sp. toads
  - DMT (dimethyltryptamine): from bark of yagé plant
- Synthetic
  - 5-MeO-DiPT, or "Foxy methoxy" (N,N-diisopropyl-5-methoxytryptamine)
  - AMT (alpha-methyltryptamine)

Toxic Dose
- Psilocybin: 40 mcg/kg
- "Foxy methoxy": 100 mg rectally reported in fatality (typical dose 10 mg)

Mechanism of Action
- Tryptamines stimulate serotonin type 2A (5HT2A) receptors to cause hallucinations

Clinical Manifestations
- CNS
  - Visual and auditory hallucinations or illusions
  - Synesthesias
  - Body dysmorphisms

FOR ALL HALLUCINOGENS/PSYCHOTROPIC AGENTS

Diagnostics
- Quantitative concentration not readily available
- Evaluation for secondary injury/trauma
- EKG
- BMP
- CPK
- Urine drug screen of abuse

> **PEARL.** Dextromethorphan/ketamine can cause false + for PCP

Treatment
- ABCDE

> **PEARL.** Reassurance and observation in a quiet, safe environment are often the only interventions required to manage a dysphoric reaction

- Agitation
  - Diazepam
    - Adult: 5-10 mg IV q5-10min PRN
    - Pediatric: 0.2-0.5 mg/kg IV q5-10min
  - Lorazepam
    - Adult: 2-4 mg IV q15min PRN
    - Pediatric: 0.05-0.1 mg/kg IV q10-15min PRN
- GI distress
  - IV fluids
  - Anti-emetics

Disposition
- Observe minimum 6 hrs
- Admit severe, persistent, or worsening signs and symptoms

MARIJUANA

Tetrahydrocannabinol (THC)

Sources
- *Cannabis sativa* plant contains cannabinoids: cannabinol, cannabidiol, and tetrahydrocannabinol (THC)
- Medicinal compounds including dronabinol and cannabidiol
- Cannabis-containing edibles
- Hash oil and other products

Toxic Dose
- Dependent on variable concentrations of Δ9-THC in cigarette or hashish

Mechanism of Action
- Δ9-THC binds to cannabinoid receptors CB1 and CB2
- CB1: Distributed throughout brain; thought to be responsible for producing the clinical effects of cannabinoid use
- CB2: Located peripherally in immune system tissues (splenic macrophages), peripheral nerve terminals

Clinical Manifestations
- ACUTE
  - Tachycardia
  - Sedation
  - Postural hypotension
  - Dysphoria
  - Paranoia
  - Symptoms may be delayed for hours after consumption of edibles
- CHRONIC

  PEARL. Cannabinoid hyperemesis
  - Recurrent episodes nausea/vomiting
  - Multiple ED visits
  - Brief relief with hot showers
  - Relief with topical capsaicin cream

Diagnostics
- Urine THC screen if indicated
  - May be detected for weeks depending on chronicity of use

  PEARL. Variable cross reactivity in urine screening reported for ibuprofen, naproxen, efavirenz, and pantoprazole

Treatment
- ABCDE
- Anxiety/paranoia
  - Diazepam
    - Adult: 5-10 mg IV q5-10min PRN
    - Pediatric: 0.2-0.5 mg/kg IV q5-10min PRN
  - Lorazepam
    - Adult: 2-4 mg IV q10-15min PRN
    - Pediatric: 0.05-0.1 mg/kg IV q10-15min PRN
  - Haloperidol
    - Adult: 2-5 mg IV/IM, repeat PRN 10-30 min
- Cannabinoid hyperemesis
  - Stop exposure, patients instructed to abstain from THC use
  - IVF
  - Symptomatic management of nausea
  - Avoid opioid use to treat abdominal pain—can elicit further vomiting

  PEARL. Capsaicin cream applied to abdomen

Disposition
- Observe minimum 6 hrs
- Admit severe, persistent, or worsening signs and symptoms

  PEARL. Children exposed to edibles may develop significant toxicity requiring admission

Synthetic Cannabinoids

Sources
- Research chemicals often sold under the guise of potpourri or incense
- "K2"
- "Spice"

Toxic Dose
- Variable; little specific human data reported

Mechanism of Action
- Full cannabinoid receptor agonist with greater binding affinity to CB1 receptors than THC
  - 2-100 times more potent than THC
  - Large class with numerous different agents all structurally unrelated to THC

Clinical Manifestations
- CNS
  - Severe agitation
  - Delirium
  - Seizure and status epilepticus
  - Coma
- CV
  - Tachycardia
  - Arrhythmia has been reported
  - Bradycardia
  - Hypertension
  - Hypotension
- Renal injury

Diagnostics

PEARL. NOT detected by routine urine drug screen testing

- BMP
- CPK
- EKG

Treatment
- ABCDE
- Agitation/Seizures
  - Diazepam
    - Adult: 5-10 mg IV q5-10min PRN
    - Pediatric: 0.2-0.5 mg/kg IV q5-10min PRN
  - Lorazepam
    - Adult: 2-4 mg IV q10-15min PRN
    - Pediatric: 0.05-0.1 mg/kg IV q10-15min PRN
  - Phenobarbital
    - 1-20 mg/kg IV over 60 min
  - Propofol (if intubated)
    - Continuous infusion of 5 mcg/kg/min and titrate (rec. max of 55 mcg/kg/min)

Disposition
- Admit severe, persistent, or worsening signs and symptoms

NICOTINE

Sources
- Nicotine products—liquids, plants, gums, transdermal patches, lozenges
- Neonicotinoid insecticides
- Tobacco harvesters

Toxic Dose
- Can occur with ingesting as little as 1 cigarette, 3 or more butts
- Can be absorbed dermally in tobacco harvesting
- Nicotine liquids can be potentially fatal in small doses

Mechanism of Action
- Mimics acetylcholine by directly stimulating nicotine receptors
- Causes release of norepinephrine, acetylcholine, GABA, serotonin, glutamate, and dopamine

Clinical Manifestations
- Initially can present with hypertension and tachycardia that will progress to hypotension and bradycardia
- Biphasic presentation: Initially central stimulation, then depression
- Respiratory arrest is most likely cause of death
- Early—nicotinic cholinergic crisis (See Toxidrome Table, p. 282)
    - Salivation
    - Tachycardia
    - N/V
    - Abdominal cramping
    - Hypertension
    - Diaphoresis
    - Seizure
- Late
    - Bradycardia
    - Lethargy and confusion
    - Coma

PEARL. Usually toxicity demonstrated within 20 min of ingestion
- Exception: transdermal patches, nicotine gums

PEARL. Consider nicotine poisoning in pediatric patient with N/V, salivation, and weakness if parents use nicotine products

Diagnostics
- BMP
- No specific test for nicotine or metabolite cotinine

Treatment
- ABCDE
- Cholinergic symptoms
  — Atropine (see above dosing)
- Seizure
  — Diazepam
    - Adult: 5-10 mg IV q5-10min PRN
    - Pediatric: 0.2-0.5 mg/kg IV q5-10min
  — Lorazepam
    - Adult: 2-4 mg IV q10-15min PRN
    - Pediatric: 0.05-0.1 mg/kg IV q10-15min PRN
  — Phenobarbital
    - 130-260 mg IV q 20min titrate to effect (in adults)
    - 10 mg/kg IVPB may require secure airway
  — Propofol (if intubated)
    - Continuous infusion of 5 mcg/kg/min titrate (rec. max of 55 mcg/kg/min)

Disposition
- Observe minimum 6 hrs
- Admit
  — Ingestion of gums, patches
  — Severe, persistent, or worsening signs and symptoms

SYMPATHOMIMETICS

Sources
- Cocaine
- Phenylethylamines
  — Cathinones
  — Amphetamines
  — 3,4-methylenedioxymethamphetamine (MDMA)

Toxic Dose
- Cocaine: Ingestion of > 1 g potentially fatal
- In general, narrow therapeutic index

Mechanism of Action
- Indirect acting α and β adrenergic receptor agonism via increased release or inhibition of catecholamine reuptake
- Cocaine
  - Blockade the reuptake of norepinephrine, serotonin, epinephrine, and dopamine

  PEARL. Causes Na^+ channel blockade (local anesthetic effect, membrane-stabilizing effect)

- Amphetamines
  - Increases release of catecholamines (norepinephrine, serotonin, dopamine) from pre-synaptic terminals
  - Blockade of norepinephrine, serotonin, and dopamine reuptake by competitive inhibition
  - Inhibition of monoamine oxidase (MOA)

Clinical Manifestations
- Sympathomimetic toxidrome (See Toxidrome Table, p. 282)
  - Diaphoresis
  - Tachycardia
  - Mydriasis
  - Hypertension
  - Hyperthermia
  - Delirium
  - Pressured speech
- CNS
  - Altered mental status
  - Seizures
- Musculoskeletal
  - Rhabdomyolysis: MDMA
- Vascular
  - Vasoconstriction
  - Vaso-occlusion
    - Stroke
    - Ischemic colitis

- CV
  - Cardiomyopathy from chronic abuse
  - Na^+ blockade (QRS prolongation): Cocaine
  - MI
- Metabolic
  - Hypokalemia
  - Metabolic acidosis
  - Hyperglycemia
  - Hyponatremia: MDMA
- Cocaine

  PEARL. When combined with ethanol, forms cocaethylene, which has longer duration of action than cocaine alone and has been associated with higher risk of sudden death

  - Barotrauma can occur following Valsalva maneuver to retain the drug (smoked and intranasal)

  PEARL. "Crack lung" is a respiratory complication when smoked. Constellation of symptoms include:

  - Fever
  - Hemoptysis
  - Hypoxia
  - ARDS
  - "Crack dancing"—choreoathetoid movements

Diagnostics
- Urine drug screen (immunoassay)
  - **Cocaine**

    PEARL. Benzoylecgonine is the cocaine metabolite identified

    - False positives are rare because of high specificity
    - May be positive for up to 3 days
  - **Amphetamine**

    PEARL. Many drugs cause false positive because of structural similarity

    - Bupropion
    - Trazodone
    - Labetalol
    - Ranitidine
    - Chlorpromazine

- BMP
- CPK
- EKG

PEARL. Cocaine may be contaminated with levamisole, which can cause agranulocytosis and vasculitis

- Differentiation from anticholinergic toxidrome
  - "Wet" (diaphoretic) as opposed to "dry" with anticholinergic
  - Speech pattern is distinct pressured vs. garbled with anticholinergic
  - See Toxidrome Table, p. 282

Treatment
- ABCDE
- Fluid resuscitation for volume depletion
- Hyperthermia
  - Aggressive cooling
  - Control excessive motor activity
- Agitation/seizures
  - Diazepam
    - Adult: 5-10 mg IV q5-10min PRN
    - Pediatric: 0.2-0.5 mg/kg IV q5-10min
  - Lorazepam
    - Adult: 2-4 mg IV q10-15min PRN
    - Pediatric: 0.05-0.1 mg/kg IV q10-15min PRN
  - Phenobarbital
    - 130-260 mg IV q20min titrate to effect (in adults)
    - 10 mg/kg IVPB may require secure airway
  - Propofol (if intubated)
    - Continuous infusion of 5 mcg/kg/min titrate (rec. max of 55 mcg/kg/min)
- If intubation is needed to control agitation or hyperthermia, avoid succinylcholine, use non-depolarizing neuromuscular blockers if hyperthermic, hyperkalemic, or have rhabdomyolysis
- Hypertension
  - Consider direct vasodilator for persistent hypertension despite sedatives
    - Phentolamine
      - Adults: 5 mg IM, IV

- ♦ Pediatrics: 0.05-0.1 mg/kg/dose IV (max 5 mg)
- ■ QRS prolongation (due to Na^+ channel blocking effects of cocaine)
  - — Sodium bicarbonate
    - • Bolus: 1-2 mEq/kg IVP over 1-2 min
    - • Infusion: 100-150 mEq in 1 L D5W @ 150-200 mL/h (2x maintenance in pediatrics)
- ■ Choreoathetosis ("crack dancing")
  - — Haloperidol
    - • Adult: 5 mg IV/IM, repeat PRN 10-30 min

Disposition

- ■ Admit severe, persistent, or worsening signs and symptoms or those requiring antidotal treatment

SPECIAL SYNDROMES

MALIGNANT HYPERTHERMIA

Source
- General anesthesia (volatile anesthetics)
- Succinylcholine

Toxic Dose
- Likely dose-dependent but minimum dose unknown

Mechanism of Action
- Genetic disorder (autosomal dominant) most commonly involving defect in the ryanodine receptor (RYR1) in skeletal muscle
- This defect results in uncontrolled Ca^{2+} release from the sarcoplasmic reticulum (SR) and the subsequent hypermetabolic response in an attempt to decrease intracellular Ca^{2+} via sequestration in the SR
- This results in increased metabolism, oxygen and ATP consumption leading to muscle rigidity and cell damage and breakdown
- MH is associated with other myopathies

Clinical Manifestations
- Signs of MH typically develop in the operating room or post-op recovery unit
- Early

    PEARL. Increase in ETCO2 (earliest most sensitive sign)

    — Tachycardia
    — Muscle rigidity
    — HTN
    — Hypoxia
    — Combined metabolic-respiratory acidosis
    — Masseter muscle rigidity
- Late

    PEARL. Hyperthermia (diagnosis typically made prior to its development)

    — Hyperkalemia
    — Rhabdomyolysis
    — Acute renal failure
    — Hypotension
    — Dysrhythmia
    — CV collapse
    — DIC

PEARL. Previous uneventful anesthetic exposure does not rule out possibility of developing malignant hyperthermia

PEARL. After malignant hyperthermia develops, neuromuscular blocking agents may not effectively induce paralysis

Diagnostics
- Monitor ETCO2
- ABG/VBG
- BMP (particularly K^+)
- CPK
- PT
- Ca^{2+}
- Genetic and confirmatory diagnostic testing available but not helpful in acute management

Treatment
- ABCDE
- Early recognition and discontinue triggering agents immediately
- Hyperventilation using mechanical ventilation (minute ventilation > 200 mL/kg/min)
- Dantrolene
  — 2.5 mg/kg IV rapidly
  — Repeat 1 mg/kg boluses q5-10min to achieve clinical response (max 10 mg/kg)
  — Administer 1 mg/kg q6hrs to prevent recurrence
    - AVOID use of calcium channel blockers, especially verapamil and dantrolene; combination causes hyperkalemia and cardiovascular collapse
- Active cooling measures
- Monitor for and treat hyperkalemia
- Sodium bicarbonate may be considered in setting of hyperkalemia, rhabdomyolysis, or severe refractory acidosis

PEARL. Call MHAUS (Malignant Hyperthermia Association of the United States hotline to assist with patient management https://www.mhaus.org/

  — **U.S. and Canada: 800-MH-HYPER (800-644-9737)**
  — **Referral of patient and family for genetic and confirmatory testing**

Disposition
- Admit all to ICU

NEUROLEPTIC MALIGNANT SYNDROME

Source
- Neuroleptic agents
- Risk factors
  - High potency antipsychotics
  - Depot formulations
  - Rapid dose escalation
  - Dehydration
  - Prior brain injury
  - Previous episode of NMS

Mechanism of Action
- Central blockade of dopamine (D2) receptors in the striatum and hypothalamus

PEARL. Typically seen in first 1-2 weeks after starting an antipsychotic

- But may be seen after recent escalation of dosage or prolonged use of antipsychotics
- Abrupt withdrawal from dopaminergic agents (Parkinson's disease)

PEARL. Onset is gradual (distinction of serotonin syndrome which is abrupt)

Clinical Manifestations (See Toxidrome Table, p. 282)

PEARL. Tetrad of altered mental status, muscular rigidity, hyperthermia and autonomic instability

  - Hyperthermia (temp > 38°C is common; may exceed 40°C)
  - Altered mental status (lethargy, catatonia, coma, agitation)
  - Autonomic instability (tachycardia, tachypnea, labile BP)
  - Muscular rigidity ("lead pipe")
  - Mutism
  - Hyperreflexia
- Complications
  - Metabolic acidosis
  - Rhabdomyolysis
  - DIC
  - Acute kidney injury
  - Cardiac dysrhythmias
  - Fluctuations in clinical manifestation may be seen
  - Aspiration pneumonia
  - DVT

Diagnostics
- BMP
- CPK
- PT
- LFT
- Neuroimaging, lumbar puncture, EEG are often unrevealing but necessary to rule out other causes
- No confirmatory test available, exclude other diagnoses

Treatment
- ABCDE

PEARL. Discontinue neuroleptic or resume dopamine agonist (Parkinson medication)

- Rapid, active cooling for goal of normal core temperature within 30 min
- Hyperthermia and motor hyperactivity
  - Diazepam
    - Adult: 5-10 mg IV q5-10min PRN
    - Pediatric: 0.2-0.5 mg/kg IV q5-10min
  - Lorazepam
    - Adult: 2-4 mg IV q15min PRN
    - Pediatric: 0.05-0.1 mg/kg IV q15min PRN
  - Phenobarbital
    - 130-260 mg IV q 20min titrate to effect (in adults)
    - 10 mg/kg IVPB likely to require secure airway
  - Propofol (if intubated)
    - Continuous infusion of 5 mcg/kg/min titrate (rec. max of 55 mcg/kg/min)
  - Consider non-depolarizing neuromuscular blockade in cases with refractory muscle hyperactivity/rigidity
  - Bromocriptine (level of evidence is poor, not routinely recommended)
    - 2.5 mg PO q8hrs
    - Monitor for recrudescence of signs of NMS on discontinuation
  - Limited evidence suggests ECT for severe prolonged cases unresponsive to maximal supportive care
- Hypotension
  - Volume expansion
  - Direct-acting vasopressors (epi, norepi)

- Treatment of anticipated complications
  - Aspiration pneumonia (airway protection, ventilation, oxygenation, antibiotics)
  - DVT/PE (anticoagulation)
  - Acute kidney injury (volume resuscitation)
  - Rhabdomyolysis (ensure adequate UOP > 1mL/kg/hr)
- Anticipated resolution within 7-14 days but can be protracted (especially with depot formulations)

Disposition
- Admit all to ICU

SEROTONIN SYNDROME

Sources
- SSRI/SNRI
- TCA
- MAOIs
- Stimulants
  - Cocaine
  - Amphetamines
  - MDMA
- Opioids
  - Meperidine
  - Dextromethorphan
  - Tramadol/tapentadol
  - *Limited evidence implicating fentanyl
- Other
  - Lithium
  - Linezolid
  - L-tryptophan
  - St. John's wort
  - Sumatriptan

Mechanism of Action
- Involves excessive stimulation of serotonin 5-HT2A/5-HT1A receptors
- Commonly from combination of serotonergic drugs but can occur with single agent at high therapeutic dose or in overdose
- Typically develops shortly after increase in dose or transitioning from one serotonergic agent to another

Clinical Manifestations

> **PEARL.** Rapid onset (within hours)

> **PEARL.** Triad of autonomic instability, altered mental status, and neuromuscular dysfunction

- Autonomic instability
  - Hyperthermia
  - Tachycardia
  - Labile blood pressure
  - Dysrhythmias
- Altered mental status
  - Delirium
  - Coma
  - Confusion
  - Anxiety
  - Agitation
  - Seizures
- Neuromuscular dysfunction
  - Clonus/myoclonus
  - Tremor
  - Hyperreflexia
  - Rigidity
    > **PEARL.** Lower extremity > upper extremity
- Other: GI
  - Diarrhea
- Complications: rhabdomyolysis, acute renal failure, elevated LFT, coagulopathy, DIC, hypotension, cardiac arrest

Diagnostics

- Diagnosis of exclusion
- No specific confirmatory test
- BMP
- CPK
- Lactate
- EKG

Treatment
- ABCDE
- Discontinue all serotonergic drug(s)
- Hyperthermia: rapid cooling (normal core temp in < 30 min)
  - Requires control of motor hyperactivity and prevention of shivering
- Agitation and motor hyperactivity
  - Diazepam
    - Adult: 5-10 mg IV q5-10min PRN
    - Pediatric: 0.2-0.5 mg/kg IV q5-10min
  - Lorazepam
    - Adult: 2-4 mg IV q15min PRN
    - Pediatric: 0.05-0.1 mg/kg IV q15min PRN
  - Phenobarbital
    - 130-260 mg IV q20min titrate to effect (in adults)
    - 10 mg/kg IVPB likely to require secure airway
  - Propofol (if intubated)
    - Continuous infusion of 5 mcg/kg/min titrate (rec. max of 55 mcg/kg/min)
- Cyproheptadine
  - Nonselective serotonin antagonist
  - Efficacy and benefits in humans with SS not substantiated
  - Use is limited because of anticholinergic effects and it is only available for oral dosing

Disposition
- Consider admitting all, especially those with severe, persistent, or worsening signs and symptoms

TOXIC INHALANTS

INHALED GAS

Chlorine

Sources
- Industrial exposure
- Transportation accidents
- Household cleaning products
  - Glass/window cleaners
  - Toilet bowl cleaners
  - Concrete/grout cleaners
  - Drain cleaners
  - Lime/rust/calcium removers
- Swimming pool
- Chemical warfare agent

Toxic Dose
- 1-3 ppm: Mild mucus membrane irritation
- 5-15 ppm: Moderate mucus membrane irritation
- > 30 ppm: Substernal chest pain, SOB, cough
- 40-60 ppm: Toxic pneumonitis/pulmonary edema
- ~400 ppm: Fatal within 30 min
- ~1000 ppm: Fatal within minutes

Mechanism of Action
- Interacts with water on mucosal surfaces to form hypochlorous acid and hydrochloric acid
- Promoting inflammatory cascade

Clinical Manifestations
- Pulmonary
  - Respiratory distress
  - Cough
  - Upper airway irritation
  - Bronchospasm
- Ophthalmologic irritation

Diagnostics
- ABG/VBG
- CXR
  - Majority unremarkable
  - Pulmonary edema
    - Massive exposure

Treatment
- Removal from exposure
- Flush irritated mucosal surfaces with water
- Decontamination: Skin or clothing, use soap and water
- Humidified supplemental oxygen
- Nebulized β2-agonists
- Severe acute lung injury may necessitate Intubation and mechanical ventilation (ARDS vent settings)
- Corticosteroids are controversial and data limited
  - Typically reserved for patients at risk for developing bronchiolitis obliterans

Disposition
- Admit severe, persistent, or worsening signs and symptoms

Hydrogen Sulfide

Sources
- Exposure commonly occurs in waste management, petroleum, natural gas industries
- Product of the decay of organic matter (ie, sewers and manure pits)
- Natural sources include volcanic eruptions and sulfur springs

> **PEARL.** Mode of suicide by mixing household products in enclosed spaces
> - "Detergent suicide" mixing a sulfur-containing product with acidic toilet bowl cleaner

Toxic Concentration
- Colorless gas denser than air with an odor of rotten eggs; exposure is through inhalation
  - 0.02-0.13 ppm: Odor threshold
  - 20-30 ppm: Intense rotten egg odor
  - 50-100 ppm: Mucous membrane irritation

- 100-150 ppm: Olfactory fatigue/loss of smell
  > **PEARL.** Rotten egg odor unreliable at high concentrations because of olfactory fatigue
- 200-300 ppm: Irritation of respiratory tract and eyes, acute lung injury
- \> 500 ppm: Systemic toxicity
- 700 ppm: "Knock down" effect, cardiopulmonary arrest, immediately fatal

Mechanism of Action
- Inhibits oxidative metabolism by binding to cytochrome c oxidase in the electron transport chain and impairing ATP production
- Mucous membrane irritant via reaction with water to form acid sulfides

Clinical Manifestations

> **PEARL.** Must maintain high clinical suspicion if patient found unresponsive, multiple victims at scene

- CNS
  - Rapid knockdown ("slaughterhouse sledgehammer effect")
  - Seizure
  - Coma
- Ophthalmologic
  - Keratoconjunctivitis ("gas eye")
  - Photophobia
  - Lacrimation
  - Pain
  - Corneal erosions and ulcerations
- Pulmonary
  - Increased respiratory rate
  - Pulmonary edema/acute lung injury
- CV
  - Tachycardia
  - Hypotension
  - Dysrhythmias, rapid CV collapse
- Metabolic acidosis

Diagnostics
- Results of atmospheric air sample monitoring devices may be useful but should be interpreted cautiously because of potential for rapid dissipation
  - May also measure CO, CO_2, O_2
- Whole blood sulfide concentration not readily available and nonspecific
  - Leaving exposure history and clinical presentation

- Odor of rotten eggs from patient or belongings

PEARL. Darkening of silver jewelry or coins on patient at time of exposure (caused by conversion to silver sulfide)

- ABG/VBG and co-oximetry (MetHb, COHb and other causes of metabolic acidosis)
- Lactate
- BMP
- EKG
- CXR/neuroimaging (secondary trauma)

Treatment
- Immediate removal from source
  - Only attempt rescue if using self-contained breathing apparatus; emergency personnel must avoid becoming secondary victims
  - Move victim to fresh air and administer 100% oxygen
- ABCDE
- High flow oxygen and mechanical ventilation
- Hypotension
  - Volume resuscitation and direct-acting vasopressors
- Metabolic acidosis
  - If severe and unresponsive to other measures, consider sodium bicarbonate
- Identify and treat secondary trauma from rapid loss of consciousness
- Ophthalmologic injury and mucous membrane irritation
  - Copious irrigation
  - Cycloplegics and ophthalmic antibiotics
- Low level evidence for antidotal therapy and considering H2S is short-lived once removed from source it is not routinely recommended
  - Sodium nitrite ($NaNO_2$) 3% 10 mL (pediatric dose: 0.33 mL/kg)
    - Contraindications: hypoxia, hypotension, or patients unable to tolerate methemoglobin formation
  - No role for sodium thiosulfate
  - Use of hydroxocobalamin, or HBO, cannot be recommended at this time based on lack of evidence

Disposition
- Admit all symptomatic patients

Nitrogen Dioxide

Sources
- Reddish, brown gas
- Welding
- Nitrocellulose combustion
- Grain silos ("Silo-filler's disease")
- Zamboni ("Ice hockey lung")

    PEARL. Ice resurfacing machines can cause toxicity from either nitrogen dioxide or carbon monoxide depending on air/fuel mixture

Toxic Dose
- 20 ppm: IDLH

Mechanism of Action
- Combines with water to form nitric and nitrous acid
- Reactive nitrous species

Clinical Manifestations
- ACUTE
    - Often asymptomatic
    - Pulmonary irritation
    - Dyspnea
    - Cough
    - Hemoptysis
    - Methemoglobinemia

    PEARL. Delayed pulmonary edema 24 hrs

- CHRONIC
    - Chronic bronchitis
    - Chronic cough

Diagnostics
- ABG/VBG
- Co-oximetry
- CXR (Pulmonary edema)

Treatment
- Removal from exposure
- Supplemental oxygen
- β2 agonists

- Consider IV corticosteroids if concerned for potential to develop bronchiolitis obliterans [limited data]
- Methylene blue if methemoglobinemia

Disposition

PEARL. Admit for all acute exposure because of delayed pulmonary edema

Phosgene

Sources
- Dyes
- Agricultural chemicals
- Synthetic foams
- Resins
- Polymers/polycarbonates for industrial use
- Chemical warfare agent

PEARL. Odor of freshly mown hay

Toxic Dose
- 3 ppm: Throat irritation
- 4 ppm: Eye irritation
- 4.8 ppm: Cough, chest tightness
- 300 ppm/min: Lethal for 50% of the population

Mechanism of Action
- Hydrolysis: Combines with water to produce hydrogen chloride and carbon dioxide
- Acylation: Phosgene loses carbon and oxygen to hydroxyl, thiol, amine, sulfhydryl groups on proteins, carbohydrates, lipids

Clinical Manifestations
- 3 phases
  - Reflex (early)
    - Eye/nose/throat irritation
  - Latency
    - Decreasing symptoms
  - Pulmonary edema (up to 48 hrs)
    - Dyspnea
    - Cough
    - Respiratory failure

Diagnostics

- CXR
  - Hilar enlargement
  - Pulmonary edema

Treatment

- Removal from source
- O_2
  - Limit to 40% FiO_2 to prevent oxygen toxicity
- Consider Ibuprofen
- Consider IV corticosteroids (limited data)
- Positive end-expiratory pressure (PEEP)
- ECMO

Disposition

PEARL. Admit for all exposures because of delayed pulmonary edema

WITHDRAWAL STATES

ETHANOL WITHDRAWAL

Sources
- Alcoholic beverages
- Hand sanitizers
- Perfumes
- Cologne

Mechanism of Withdrawal
- Acute decrease/discontinuation of consumption of alcohol
- Central nervous system hyperexcitation
  - Decrease in inhibitory $GABA_A$
  - Increase in excitatory glutamate at NMDA receptor

Clinical Manifestations
- Alcoholic tremulousness
  - Onset 6-24 hrs after decrease/cessation
  - Autonomic hyperactivity
    - Tachycardia
    - Hypertension

  PEARL. Tremor (tongue fasciculations most sensitive)

    - Anxiety
    - Diaphoresis
    - Nausea
- Alcoholic hallucinosis
  - Tactile (most common)
  - Visual

  PEARL. Preserved sensorium if isolated hallucinosis, although hallucinations can complicate classic alcohol withdrawal

- Seizures
  - Can be presenting sign of alcohol withdrawal
  - May occur in absence of other features of alcohol withdrawal
  - Generalized, brief, tonic-clonic
  - Short postictal period
  - Status/focal seizures atypical
  - 33% develop Delirium Tremens

- Delirium tremens
  - Onset 48-96 hrs, potential for prolonged duration
  - Altered consciousness or cognition
  - Autonomic hyperactivity
  - Psychomotor agitation
  - Associated morbidity and mortality if unrecognized and untreated

Diagnostics
- Clinical diagnosis no diagnostic test confirms or predicts ethanol withdrawal
- Most reliable predictor is previous history of ethanol withdrawal
- Serum ethanol concentration is not prognostic

    PEARL. Ethanol withdrawal can occur with detectable concentration

- CBC
  - Macrocytosis
  - Thrombocytopenia
- BMP
  - Hyponatremia
  - Hypokalemia
  - Hypomagnesemia
  - Alcoholic ketoacidosis (AG metabolic acidosis)
  - Contraction alkalosis
- LFT
  - Transaminitis
    - 2:1 AST/ALT
  - Hyperbilirubinemia
- Lactate
  - Lactemia
    - Can be markedly elevated in setting of AKA
- CT head

    PEARL. Perform in cases of seizures or possible trauma, or patients found unresponsive with no available history

PEARL. Ethanol withdrawal is a clinical diagnosis; therefore, always consider other etiologies of clinical presentation; evaluate for underlying illness prompting cessation from alcohol use

Treatment
- See algorithm, p. 263
- D5 IVF as clinically indicated
- Correct hypoglycemia
- Vitamin supplementation
  - Thiamine
  - Preferentially excreted/malabsorbed in alcoholics
  - Prevent precipitating/worsening Wernicke's encephalopathy

    PEARL. Unnecessary to administer before glucose if patient hypoglycemic

    - 500 mg IV TID if treating Wernicke's encephalopathy
    - 200-500 mg IV for suspected thiamine deficiency
    - 100 mg is sufficient to prevent thiamine deficiency
  - MVI IV/PO
  - Folate
    - 1 mg IV/PO
- Electrolyte replacement as indicated
- Mild withdrawal
  - Patients often self-manage symptoms with alcohol
  - Consider short oral benzodiazepine taper
    - Lorazepam
      - 2-4 mg PO q6hrs
    - Diazepam
      - 10-20 mg PO q8hrs
    - Chlordiazepoxide
      - 50-100 mg PO q6hrs
- Moderate to severe withdrawal
  - IV benzodiazepines
    - Rapidly escalating doses
  - Dose to achieve vital sign improvement and mild sedation (eg, lid lag)
  - Diazepam (preferred initial agent)
    - Lipophilic, rapid effect
    - Active metabolites
    - 10, 20, 40, 80, 100 mg IV q5-10min per dose PRN titrated to effect in doubling doses
  - Lorazepam
    - May be preferred agent in those with severe liver disease or elderly
    - 2, 4, 8, 16 mg IV q15-20min per dose PRN

- IV phenobarbital
  - 130-260 mg IV q20min
  - Consider in those resistant to benzodiazepines
  - Higher risk respiratory depression and hypotension when larger doses used
- Alcohol withdrawal refractory to benzodiazepines
  - IV phenobarbital load 10-20 mg/kg IVPB may require secured airway
  - IV propofol 5 mcg/kg/min can be used as adjunct in intubated patients
  - IV ketamine can be considered as adjunct therapy
    - 0.3 mg/kg/h or 1-1.5 mg/kg IV
  - Avoid haloperidol alone for agitation as does not address underlying pathophysiology and lowers seizure threshold

Disposition
- See algorithm, p. 263
- Discharge
  - Not intoxicated, normal vital signs
  - Consider social support and ability to comply with outpatient therapies
  - No significant underlying medical or psychiatric acute illness
- Inpatient medical or detoxification unit
  - Improved vital signs
  - No significant underlying surgical or medical condition requiring ICU-level care
  - Clear sensorium
  - Tolerates 2-4 hrs between doses of benzodiazepines
  - Responsive to 10-20 mg diazepam or equivalent
- ICU
  - Delirium tremens
  - Frequent or high doses of medications to control symptoms
  - History of complicated alcohol withdrawal

Clinical Pathway for Emergency Department Management of Alcohol Withdrawal Syndrome

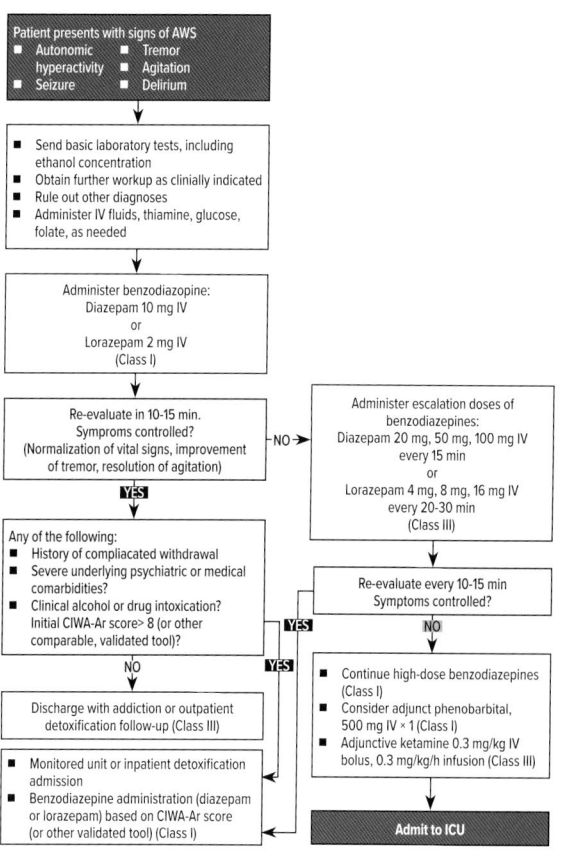

OPIOID WITHDRAWAL

Mechanism of Withdrawal
- Cessation of chronic opioid use
- Administration of an opioid receptor antagonist

Clinical Manifestations
- Short-acting opioids (eg, heroin, morphine)
  - First symptoms appear 6-12 hrs after last use; peak at 1-3 days and can last up to 5-6 days
- Long-acting opioids (eg, methadone)
  - First symptoms appear 36-48 hrs after last use; peak 5-6 days and can last up to 2 weeks
- CNS
  - Lacrimation
  - Yawning
  - Rhinorrhea
  - Sweating
  - Piloerection
  - Dysphoria, restlessness
  - Tremor
- GI
  - N/V/D
- Musculoskeletal
  - Bone/joint aches

PEARL. Sensorium is preserved, so altered mental status should prompt evaluation for alternative diagnosis

  - An exception is acute iatrogenic withdrawal from administration of IV opioid antagonist which may precipitate altered mental status

PEARL. Neonatal abstinence syndrome: poor feeding, irritability, seizure

Diagnostics
- Clinical diagnosis, no specific test
- Clinical Opiate Withdrawal Scale (COWS)

Treatment
- Opioid withdrawal is considered non-life-threatening except in neonates
- ABCDE
- Treatment for opioid dependence is medication-assisted therapy with buprenorphine or methadone

- Buprenorphine induction
  - May be initiated in ED but requires DATA 2000 waiver and follow-up care with an eligible prescriber
- Adjunctive treatment
  - No habituating medications should be prescribed (eg, benzodiazepines)
  - Clonidine
    - α2-adrenergic agonists have been shown to be effective in suppressing many of the autonomic symptoms of withdrawal
    - Subjective symptoms of lethargy, restlessness, insomnia, and cravings are NOT well controlled
    - Clonidine 0.1-0.3 mg PO q4hrs
  - NSAIDs for bone/joint aches (ibuprofen 600 mg PO q6hrs)
  - Anti-emetics (eg, ondansetron)
  - Trazodone 50-100 mg PO PRN insomnia
  - Hydroxyzine 25-50 mg PO q6hrs insomnia/restlessness
  - GI complaints
    - Antiemetic/antidiarrheal
  - Loperamide

    PEARL. High-dose loperamide abuse associated with QT prolongation and torsades de pointes (See Loperamide, p. 186)

- Consider naloxone prescription at discharge
- Referral or enrollment in substance use disorder treatment program
- Non-cardiogenic pulmonary edema
  - Setting of rapid reversal with naloxone but likely opioid toxicity itself
  - Oxygen
  - CPAP

Disposition
- Admit severe, persistent, or worsening signs and symptoms

SEDATIVE/HYPNOTIC WITHDRAWAL (SEE TOXIDROME TABLE, APPENDIX)

Sources
- Benzodiazepines: $GABA_A$ receptor agonists (See Benzodiazepines, p. 195)
  - Alprazolam
  - Diazepam
  - Lorazepam
- Barbiturates: $GABA_A$ receptor agonists (See Barbiturates, p. 193)
  - Phenobarbital
  - Butalbital

- Ethanol (See Ethanol, p. 9, and Ethanol Withdrawal, p. 259)
- GABA$_B$ receptor agonists
  — Baclofen (See Baclofen, p. 197)
  — Gamma-hydroxybutyric acid (GHB) (See GHB, p. 199)
  — Gamma-butyrolactone (GBL)
  — 1,4 Butane-diol (1,4 BD)
- Non-benzodiazepine sedative/hypnotics
  — Zolpidem (See Z Drugs, p. 200)
  — Carisoprodol (See Sedatives & Hypnotics, p. 196)

Mechanism of Withdrawal

- Chronic exposure leads to drug-induced neuroadaptations
  — Down-regulation of GABA receptors, changes in receptor subunit expression
  — Up-regulation of NMDA receptors
- Abrupt withdrawal of the agent results in:
  — Increased excitatory glutamate NMDA neurotransmission produces CNS excitation seen with withdrawal
  — Decreased inhibitory GABA neurotransmission

Clinical Manifestations

- Common onset/duration
  — Alprazolam: within 24-48 hrs; can last 4-5 days
  — Lorazepam: within 2-4 days; can last weeks
  — Diazepam: within 5-7 days; lasting weeks
  — GHB/GBL: within 1-4 hrs; lasting 3-5 days
  — Butalbital: within 4-6 hrs; lasting 3-5 days
  — Phenobarbital: within 5-7 days; lasting 3-5 days
  — Carisoprodol: within 12-48 hrs; lasting days
  — CV
    - Peripheral hyperadrenergic signs
    - Tachycardia
    - Hypertension
  — CNS
    - Altered mental status, hallucinations
    - Headaches
    - Tremors
    - Seizures
    - Delirium

- Baclofen withdrawal (beware of paralyzed patients with pumps)
  — Onset: Orally: 1-2 days after cessation, Intrathecally: 12-24 hrs after cessation; symptoms can be severe and life-threatening

  PEARL. Always interrogate baclofen pumps in patients with possible toxicity or withdrawal, which can both present with seizures

  — CV
    - Hypertension
    - Tachycardia
    - Hyperthermia
    - Multi-organ dysfunction
  — CNS
    - Confusion
    - Muscle spasticity
  — Musculoskeletal
    - Rhabdomyolysis

Diagnostics
- No specific test
- Intrathecal baclofen concentration via pump interrogation

Treatment
- ABCDE

PEARL. Consider re-administration of agent from which patient withdrawing. **NOTE:** Evaluate each case individually: substance prescribed or illicit? Can a longer-acting substitute be used that makes long-term treatment optimal and safer for patient?

- Diazepam
  — Adult: 5-10 mg IV q5-10min PRN
  — Pediatric: 0.2-0.5 mg/kg IV q5-10min
- Lorazepam
  — Adult: 2-4 mg IV q15-20min PRN
  — Pediatric: 0.05-0.1 mg/kg IV q15-20min PRN
- Phenobarbital
  — 130-260 mg IV q 20min titrate to effect (in adults)
  — 10 mg/kg IVPB likely to require secure airway
- Propofol (if intubated)
  — Continuous infusion of 5 mcg/kg/min titrate (rec. max of 55 mcg/kg/min)

Disposition
- Admit
  - Severe, persistent, or worsening signs and symptoms
    - Generally most patients will need admission unless signs and symptoms are very mild, easily controlled in the ED, and good outpatient plan established

APPENDICES

COMMON FORMULAS & MNEMONICS

Anion Gap = [Na$^+$] – [Cl-] – [HCO3-] = **8-12 mEq/L**

- **M**: Methanol, Methylxanthines, Metformin
- **U**: Uremia
- **D**: Depakote (valproic acid), Dintrophenol (DNP)
- **S**: Salicylates, Hydrogen Sulfide, Seizure, SGLT2 inhibitors
- **P**: Paracetamol (5-oxoprolene), Propylene glycol, Pentavalent Arsenic
- **I**: Isoniazid, Iron, Ibuprofen
- **C**: Carbon monoxide, Cyanide
- **E**: Ethanol, Ethylene glycol

Non-Anion Gap Metabolic Acidosis

- **H**: Hyperalimentation
- **A**: Acetazolamide/topiramate
- **R**: Renal tubular acidosis, toluene
- **D**: Diarrhea
- **U**: Ureterosigmoid fistula
- **P**: Pancreatic fistula

Narrow or Negative Anion Gap

- Bromide, Iodide
- Lithium

Osmol Gap < 10 = Measured Serum Osmolality— Calculated Serum Osmolality

> **PEARL.** Calculated Osmolality = 2[Na$^+$] + [Glucose]/18 + [BUN]/2.8 + [ETOH]/4.6

- Causes of an Elevated Osmol Gap
  - Alcohols
  - Glycols
  - Ketoacids
  - Chronic Renal Failure not on HD
- Estimating the concentration of serum alcohol or glycol
  - Acetone: Osmol gap × 5.8
  - Ethanol: Osmol gap × 4.6
  - Ethylene glycol: Osmol gap × 6.2

- Isopropyl alcohol: Osmol gap × 6
- Methanol: Osmol gap × 3.2
- Propylene glycol: Osmol gap × 7.6

DRUG/ANTIDOTE APPENDIX

Atropine
- Indication: Organophosphate, carbamate, or nicotine poisoning
  - Adult: 1-2 mg (mild) or 3-5 mg (severe) IV. Double q3-5min until dry
    - Maintenance 10-20% of load IV qh, titrate PRN
  - Pediatric: 0.05-0.1 mg/kg (min 0.1 mg) IV. Double the dose if previous does not induce atropinization
- β-blocker/calcium channel blocker, α-2 agonists
  - Adult: 0.5 mg q3-5min
  - Pediatric: 0.02 mg/kg IV (minimum dose 0.1 mg when > 5 kg, max doses 0.5 mg) q3-5min

BAL—Dimercaprol
- Indication: Lead encephalopathy

  CAUTION. Dosing has been described in mg/m2 *AND* mg/kg (75 mg/m2~4 mg/kg; 50 mg/m2~3 mg/kg)

  CAUTION. in peanut allergy/hepatic insufficiency (except in cases of post arsenical jaundice)/patients with glucose-6-phosphate dehydrogenase (G6PD) deficiency

    - Deep IM only 4 mg/kg (75 mg/m2) given alone in the 1st dose and then q4h in combination with CaNa2EDTA administered at a separate site
    - Should precede CaNa2EDTA by 4 hrs
- Indication: Inorganic and mercury vapor poisoning
  - 5 mg/kg IM once
  - 2.5 mg/kg IM every 8-12 hrs for 1 day
  - Then 2.5 mg/kg IM every 12-24 hrs for 7 days

Black widow antivenom
- Indication: Severe black widow envenomation
  - Pretreat with diphenhydramine and an H2 blocker
  - 1 vial (2.5 mL) reconstituted in 10-50 mL of saline and given IV over 15 min. A second dose may be necessary in some cases.

    CAUTION. Anaphylaxis especially with known allergy to horse protein

Bromocriptine
- Indication: Neuroleptic Malignant Syndrome
  - Adult: 2.5-10 mg PO 3-4 times/day (max 45 mg)

Calcium (Elemental Ca content in 1 g CaCl = 3 g CaGluconate)
- Indication: Calcium channel blocker, systemic hydrofluoric acid poisoning
  - Adult: CaCl 10% (1 g) IV over 10-15 min; CaGluconate 10% (3 g) IV over 5-10 min CENTRAL LINE ONLY
  - Pediatric: CaCl 10% 20 mg/kg IV over 10-15 min; CaGluconate 10% 20-50 mg/kg IV over 5-10 min, not to exceed adult dose
  - Adult Infusion: 20-50 mg/kg/hr of $CaCl_2$ (10%), or 60-150 mg/kg/hr CaGluconate (10%)
- Indication: Hydrofluoric Acid
  - Dermal: 3.5 g CaGluconate plus 5 oz water-soluble lubricant

Calcium EDTA (edetate calcium disodium)
- Indication: Lead poisoning

  CAUTION. Do NOT confuse calcium EDTA with sodium EDTA (edetate disodium)
  - Lead encephalopathy: Adult/pediatric: 1500 mg/m^2/day starting 4 hrs after initial dose of dimercaprol, max 3 g/day
    - Dose must be adjusted in patients with impaired renal function
  - Dimercaprol MUST be administered 4 hrs prior because calcium EDTA, used alone, may aggravate symptoms in patients with very high blood lead levels
  - Because calcium EDTA increases renal excretion of lead, anuria is a relative contraindication

CroFab® antivenom
- Indication: Crotalid envenomation
  - Adults: 4-6 vials diluted in 250 mL NSS and administered IV over 1 hr for "control" (8-12 vials if in shock or serious active bleed)
  - Pediatric: Antivenom dosage based on venom load and severity of symptoms—NOT on patient size (refer to adult dosing)
  - Administer IV over 60 min at 25-50 mL/hr for first 10 min. If no allergic reaction is observed, increase to 250 mL/hr. Be prepared to manage anaphylactic reactions
  - Repeat PRN based on "control":
    - Laboratory values
    - Clinical examination (worsening edema, pain)
  - 2 vials IV q6hrs × 3 doses for maintenance

Cyanide antidote kit (Hope Nithiodote™ kit)
- Indication: Cyanide poisoning
  - Sodium nitrite (NaNO$_2$) 3% (30 mg/mL)
    - Adult: 300 mg IV over 2-4 min
    - Pediatric: ~6 mg/kg IV over 2-4 min (max 300 mg)
  - Sodium thiosulfate 25% (250 mg/mL)
    - Adult: 50 mL (12.5 g) IV over 10-30 min
    - Pediatric: 250-500 mg/kg IV (max 12.5 g)

WARNING. No nitrite if smoke/fire victim/CO exposure

Deferoxamine
- Indication: Acute iron toxicity
- 5 mg/kg/hr IV increasing over 15 min to 15 mg/kg/hr, max 6 g/day

Dextrose
- Indication: Hypoglycemia
  - 0.5-1.0 g/kg, adjust based on size
    - Adult: D50 (0.5 g/mL) IV
    - Pediatric: D25 (0.25 g/mL) IV
    - Neonates: D10 (0.1 g/mL) IV
    - IV dextrose infusion
      - D5W or D10W titrated to maintain euglycemia
    - Consider administering thiamine if deficient

Diazepam
- Ethanol withdrawal
  - 5-10 mg IV, q10-20min
  - May require increasing dose 20 mg -> 40 mg -> 60 mg IV
- Agitation/seizures
  - Adult: 5-10 mg IV q5-10min PRN
  - Pediatric: 0.2-0.5 mg/kg IV q5-10min PRN

Digoxin specific FAB (DigiFab®)
- Indication: Digoxin and cardiotoxic steroid poisoning
  - IV over 30 min (IVP if critical)
  - Amount ingested known: # vials = [amount mg)] × 0.8 / 0.5 mg
  - Concentration known: # vials = [level (ng/mL)] × [weight (kg)] / 100
  - Unknown ingestion/concentration (empiric therapy)
- Adult: 10 vials (acute); 3-6 vials (chronic)
- Pediatric: 1-2 vials

Dopamine
- Indication: α-2 agonist or Na⁺ opener bradycardia/hypotension
  - Adult/Peds: 5 μg/kg/min IV, increase PRN 5-10 g/kg/min q10min to max 50 g/kg/min

Epinephrine
- Indication: Shock
  - Epinephrine
    - Infusion: 0.05 mcg/kg/min. Titrate by 0.05-0.2 mcg/kg/min q15min to goal MAP. Dose range 0.5 mcg/min
    - No true max and higher dosing may be required

Esmolol
- Indication: Methylxanthine poisoning
  - Initiate @ 50 mcg/kg/min IV. Titrate by 50 mcg/kg/min q4min to goal BP/HR (max 200 mcg/kg/min)
  - Emergent onset of effect may necessitate loading dose (500 mcg/kg/min over 1-2 min)

Ethanol (EtOH)
- Indication: Methanol, ethylene glycol poisoning (note: must be compounded by pharmacy since not commercially available)
  - IV: 10% EtOH (100 mg/mL) Load: 0.8 g/kg (8 mL/kg) over 1 hr
  - Maintenance: 80-130 mg/kg/hr (0.8-1.3 mL/kg/hr)
    - Chronic alcoholism: 150 mg/kg/h (1.5 mL/kg/hr)
  - HD: 250-350 mg/kg/hr (2.5-3.5 mL/kg/hr)
  - Pediatric: Same as adult

Flumazenil (Romazicon®)
- Indication: Benzodiazepine poisoning (pediatric, naïve, or iatrogenic ONLY)
  - Adult: Initial: 0.2 mg IV
    May repeat with 0.3 mg, then 0.5 mg
  - Pediatric: 0.01 mg/kg IV up to 0.2 mg IV over 15 seconds
    - Repeat q1min × 4 dose as needed (up to total cumulative dose 0.5 mg/kg or 1 mg—whichever lower)

Folate (folic acid)
- Indication: Methanol poisoning
  - 1-2 mg/kg (50-75 mg) q4-6hr × 24 hrs
  - Extra dose at completion of hemodialysis

Fomepizole (Antizol®)

- Indication: Methanol, ethylene glycol/propylene glycol poisoning
  — Load: 15 mg/kg IV in 100 mL NS × 30 min
  — Maintenance: 10 mg/kg IV q12hrs × 4 doses, then 15 mg/kg q12hrs until concentration < 20 mg/dL
  — Hemodialysis: Give load if > 6hrs since latest dose
    - Maintenance q4hrs during HD
    - At end, give scheduled dose if > 3hrs
    - Or, ½ dose if 1-3hrs since latest dose
  — Pediatric: Same as adult

GI Decontamination

- Gastric lavage
  — Adult: 36-40 Fr
  — Pediatric: No less than 22 Fr
    - Consider airway protection
    - Rarely indicated
    - Contraindications: Caustics, large or sharp foreign body, can't protect airway, toxin not in stomach
- Activated charcoal
  — Dose: 1 g/kg PO, ideally 10:1 charcoal:drug
  — Consider in recent (1-2 hr) ingestion of toxic substance that adsorbs to charcoal and lack of contraindications (caustics, AMS, vomiting, decreased GI motility)
- Whole bowel irrigation
  — Mechanical bulk cleansing of GI tract with polyethylene glycol solution
  — Consider for ingestions with delayed/prolonged absorption, or body packers
  — Adult: 2 L/hr PO (+/- NGT, antiemetic)
  — Pediatric: 25 mL/kg/hr PO
  v. Continue until rectal effluent is clear

Glucagon

- Indication: β-blocker poisoning
  — Adult: 50 mcg/kg (max 10 mg) IV over 1-2 min, q10-15min 1-2 times PRN, then 1-5 mg/h (max 10 mg/h) IV in D5W
  — Pediatric: 50 mcg/kg IV load, then 70 mcg/kg/hr

Haloperidol
- Indication: Agitation secondary to hallucinogens or excessive dopaminergic activity (eg, "crack dancing")
  - Adult: 5 mg IV/IM, repeat PRN 10-30 min

High-dose Insulin Euglycemia (HIE)
- Indication: Calcium channel blocker or β-blocker poisoning
  - Dextrose: ± 25-50 g (0.5-1 g/kg) IV bolus, then 0.25-0.5 g/kg/h IV infusion
  - Insulin: 1 U/kg IV bolus, then 0.5-1.0 U/kg/hr IV infusion
    - Increase if no effect in 15 min
    - Titrate to 10 U/kg/hr
    - Check capillary glucose q30min initially

Hydroxocobalamin (Cyanokit®)
- Indication: Cyanide poisoning
  - 5 g IV, may repeat × 1
  - Pediatrics: 70 mg/kg (max 5 g) IV over 30 min

Intravenous Lipid Emulsion (ILE)
- Indication: Local anesthetic toxicity (LAST) and lipophilic drug toxicity
  - Loading dose 1.5 mL/kg 20% solution over 1 min
    - May repeat for persistent dysrhythmias
  - Infusion: 0.25 mL/kg/min for 3 min
- If beneficial response, continue infusion at 0.025 mL/kg/min
  - Infusion may be increased if BP declines
  - Max dose 10 mL/kg

Isoproterenol (Isuprel®)
- Indication: Torsades de pointes
- Initiate @ 5 mcg/min Titrate by 1 mcg/min q5min to goal BP/HR
- Usual MD 2-10 mcg/min; higher dosing described and may be required
- Onset < 1 min/duration ~ 10 min

Ketamine
- Indication: Ethanol withdrawal
  - 0.3 mg/kg IV bolus f/b 0.3 m/kg/hr IV

L-carnitine
- Indication: Hyperammonemia from valproic acid poisoning
- Loading dose: 100 mg/kg IV (max 6 g) over 15-30 min, then 15 mg/kg (max 3 g per dose) IV q4hrs over 10-30 min
- Prophylaxis: 100 mg/kg/d PO divided q6hrs (max 3 g/day in adults and 2 g/day in children)

Leucovorin (Folinic Acid)
- Indication: Methotrexate poisoning
  — Dose: Estimate dosing based on known MTX plasma concentration, OR 100 mg/m2 IV over 15-30 min (max 160 mg/min) q3-6hrs × several days or until serum MTX < 10 nmol/L or < 100 nmol (in cancer) and no bone marrow toxicity

Lidocaine
- Indication: Na^+ channel blocker poisoning with QRS prolongation, ventricular arrhythmias, hypotension
  — Adult: 1-1.5 mg/kg IV x1 over 2 min; repeat 0.5 to 0.75 mg/kg bolus q5-10min. Follow by infusion = 1-4 mg/min; titrate by 1-2 mg/min q10min. After 24 hrs continuous infusion, decrease infusion rate by 50%. Reduce dose in patients with CHF, shock, or hepatic disease. Max = 4 mg/min
  — Pediatric: 1 mg/kg/dose; follow with continuous IV infusion 20-50 mcg/kg/minute. May administer second bolus if delay between initial bolus and start of infusion is > 15 min. Do not exceed 20 mcg/kg/min in patients with shock, hepatic disease, cardiac arrest, or CHF

Lorazepam
- Indication: Ethanol withdrawal/agitation/seizures
  — Adult: 2-4 mg IV q10-15min PRN
  — Pediatric: 0.05-0.1 mg/kg IV q10-15min PRN

Magnesium Sulfate
- Indication: Hypomagnesemia/hypokalemia, torsades de pointes
  — Adult: 2-4 g IVPB
  — Pediatric: 20-50 mg/kg IVPB, max dose 2 g

Methylene Blue
- Indication: Methemoglobinemia
  — IV: 1-2 mg/kg (0.1-0.2 mL/kg of 1%) over 5 min q4hrs (max 7 mg/kg)

N-acetylcysteine (Acetadote®)
- Indication: Acetaminophen toxicity, aluminum phosphide poisoning
  - Oral dosing
    - 140 mg/kg load, then 70 mg/kg q4hrs for 17 doses
  - IV dosing
    - Load: 150 mg/kg for 60 min, then 50 mg/kg for 4 hrs (12.5 mg/kg/hr). Then 100 mg/kg for 16 hrs (6.25 mg/kg/hr)
  - If on HD: double dose during HD with additional ½ load when HD > 6 hrs

Naloxone (Narcan®)
- Indication: Opioid poisoning
  - Adult: Start at 0.04-0.4 mg IV/IM/SQ/IN/IO; repeat dose if initial response not adequate, up to 10 mg total. Titrate to RR ≥ 12 and sufficient tidal volume. If opioid naive, can start with 0.4 mg
  - Pediatric: 0.01 mg/kg IV (IM, SQ, IO, Intratracheal can be used but not preferred) if opioid naïve; (0.001 mg/kg if opioid dependent)
    - Titrate to 0.1 mg/kg IV if no effect
  - Neonate: (asphyxia neonatorum) 0.01 mg/kg via umbilical vein (IM, SQ) q2-3min
    For recurrent respiratory depression consider infusion: 2/3 of reversal dose infused hourly

Norepinephrine (LEVOPHED™)
- Indication: Shock
  - Infusion: 0.05 mcg/kg/min then titrate to goal MAP
  - Dosage range varies greatly depending on clinical situation
  - No true max and higher dosing may be required

Octreotide (SANDOSTATIN®)
- Indication: Sulfonylurea poisoning
  - Adult: 50 mcg SQ/IV q6hrs
  - Pediatric: 1.25 mcg/kg (max 50 mcg) SQ q6hrs

Penicillamine
- Indication: Copper or lead toxicity
- Can cause severe hematologic, renal, dermatologic adverse effects
  - Adults 250 mg QID PO for 1-2 weeks
  - Pediatric 20-30 mg/kg/daily in 4 divided doses, max 250/dose
    - Alternatively: 10-15 mg/kg/d, administered in 3-4 divided doses
    - For lead poisoning, American Academy of Pediatrics recommends use only when unacceptable ADR to both succimer and CaNa2EDTA and chelation still indicated

Prothrombin complex concentrate (PCC)
- Note: PCC is dosed based on the factor IX (FIX) component
- Direct factor Xa inhibitors: Activated PCC (FEIBA) 50 units FIX/kg IV or 4-factor PCC (Kcentra®) 50 units FIX/kg IV—various dose strategies described; none proven
- Vitamin K antagonists (warfarin): 4-factor PCC (Kcentra®)—various dose strategies exist; none proven superior
  — Pre-treatment INR 2-4: 25 units FIX/kg (max 2500)
  — Pre-treatment INR 4-6: 35 units FIX/kg (max 3500)
  — Pretreatment INR > 6: 50 units FIX/kg (max 5000)
  — Administration rate: Kcentra® (note: contains heparin): Administer reconstituted IV at a rate of 0.12 mL/kg/min (~3 units/kg/min) up to a maximum rate of 8.4 mL/min (~210 units/min)
  — FEIBA: Infuse IV at a rate not to exceed 2 units/kg/min

Phenobarbital
- Indication: Ethanol withdrawal/seizures/agitation
  — 10-20 mg/kg IV
  — > 10 mg/kg IVPB may require secure airway

Phentolamine
- Indication: Severe hypertension secondary to stimulants (eg, cocaine), black widow envenomation
  — Adults: 5 mg IM/IV
  — Pediatric: 0.05 to 0.1 mg/kg IV (max 5 mg)

Phenylephrine (Neo-Synephrine™)
- Indication: Shock
- Initiate @ 100-180 mcg/min, then titrate by 20 mcg/min q10min to goal BP
- Maximum rate (range): Infusion rates as high as 9 mcg/kg/min have been reported when treating septic shock
- Onset < 1 min / duration ~ 15-20 min

Physostigmine (Antilirium™)
- Indication: Severe anticholinergic toxicity

WARNING. Prolonged QRS, < 120 ms, NO bronchospasm or seizure
- Adult: 1-2 mg IV over > 5 min
- May repeat in 5-10 min PRN × 1-2 doses
- Pediatric: 0.02 mg/kg (max 0.5 mg) as above

Potassium Iodide
- Indication: Radioactive iodine poisoning
  - Adults and adolescents of adult size: 130 mg PO daily
  - Adolescents and children 3-18 years: 65 mg PO daily
  - Toddlers 1 month-3 years: 32 mg PO daily
  - Neonates 0-1 month: 16 mg PO daily
  - Duration of therapy may be from 1 day to many weeks, depending on public health recommendations

Protamine Sulfate
- Indication: Heparin poisoning
- 1 mg (max 50 mg) neutralizes 100 U heparin, or 100 anti-Xa U of dalteparin/tinzaparin, or 1 mg of enoxaparin
- Load: 1 mg/100 anti-Xa U IV over > 10 min
- Then: 0.5 mg/100 anti-Xa U if still bleeding

2-PAM (pralidoxime chloride)
- Indication: Organophosphate poisoning
  - Adult: 1-2 g (20-40 mg/kg) in 100 mL NS IV over 15-30 min
    - Maintenance: 8-10 mg/kg/hr or 500 mg/hr IV
  - Pediatric: 20-50 mg/kg (max 2 gm) in 100 mL NS IV × 30-60 min
    - Maintenance: 10-20 mg/kg/hr IV

Propofol
- Indication: Agitation/seizures
  - Must be intubated
  - Continuous infusion of 5 mcg/kg/min and titrate (rec. max of 55 mcg/kg/min)

Prussian Blue (Radiogardase®)
- Indication: Thallium and cesium poisoning
  - Adult: 3 g PO TID
  - Pediatric: 1 g PO TID

Pyridoxine (Vitamin B6)
- Indication: Ethylene glycol poisoning
  - Adult: 50 mg IV/IM q6hrs until intoxication resolved
- Indication: Isoniazid or gyromitrin poisoning
  - Known ingestion amount: 1 g per g of INH IV (max 5 g) Unknown: 70 mg/kg IV (max 5 gm)
    - Infuse at 0.5 g/min until seizure stops
    - Remainder IV over 4-6 hrs

Sea Snake Antivenom

- Indication: Sea snake envenomation
- Initially 1 ampule (1000 units) diluted up to 1:10 in sodium chloride over 20-30 min IV
    - Usual dose is 1-3 ampules depending on severity and rapidity of envenoming; however up to 10 have been used
    - If Sea Snake AV not available, Tiger Snake AV may be used, noting 1 vial Sea Snake is equivalent roughly to 2-4 vials of Tiger Snake AV
    - If neither Sea Snake nor Tiger Snake AV is available, Polyvalent snake AV may be considered

Scorpion Immune F(ab')$_2$ (Equine) Injection (Anascorp®)

- Indication: Severe bark scorpion envenomation
    - 3 vials reconstituted/diluted and infused IV over 10 min. Repeat 1 vial IV over 10 min q30-60min PRN

> **CAUTION.** Anaphylaxis especially with known allergy to horse protein

Sodium Bicarbonate (NaHCO$_3$)

- Indication: Na$^+$ channel blocker poisoning with QRS prolongation, metabolic acidosis, salicylate poisoning
    - 8.4% 50 mL ampule = 50 mEq
    - 7.5% 50 mL ampule = 44.6 mEq
    - Bolus: 1-2 mEq/kg IVP over 1-2 min
    - Infusion: 100-150 mEq in 1 L D5W @ 150-200 mL/h (2x maintenance in pediatrics)

Stonefish Antivenom

- Indication: Stonefish envenomation with clinical evidence of envenomation (eg, cardiac failure). May have a role in the treatment of bullrout, lionfish, and cobbler stings
- Increased risk of anaphylaxis with previous treatment
- Dosing:
    - IM: 1 ampule for every 2 spine puncture wounds (max 3 ampules)
    - IV: Dilute 1 ampule in 100 mL NS and infuse over 20 min
    - Repeat 1 ampule at a time until resolution of local and systemic features

Succimer

- Indication: Heavy metal poisoning
    - Adult and pediatric: 10 mg/kg PO q8hrs × 5 days; then q12hrs × 14 days (max 500 mg/dose)

Thiamine
- Indication: Ethanol withdrawal
  - 250-500 mg IV TID-QD up to 1000 mg in 12 hrs
- Indication: Ethylene glycol poisoning
  - 100 mg IV QD

Vitamin K1 (Phytonadione)
- Indication: warfarin/superwarfarin poisoning
- Adult: 25-50 mg PO TID-QID × 1-2 days, then per INR
- Pediatric: 5-10 mg (0.4 mg/kg/dose) BID-QID × 1-2 days, then per INR

Toxidrome Table

Toxidrome	Common Examples	Onset	Key Clinical Features	Treatment
Anticholinergic	TCAs, Antihistamines, Antipsychotics, Atropine, Jimson Weed	Hours	Mad as hatter, dry as bone, hot as hare, red as a beet, blind as a bat, full as a flask	IVF Benzodiazepines **Physostigmine**
Cholinergics	Nicotine, organophosphates, carbamates, *Clitocybe* mushrooms	Minutes to hours	**SLUDGE/DUMBELS Paralysis Seizures**	Atropine Glycopyrrolate 2-PAM (OP)
GABA/Sedative-hypnotic withdrawal	Ethanol, benzodiazepines, **carisoprodol, baclofen**	Hours-days depending on drug (alprazolam vs. clonazepam)	Tachycardia, hypertension delirium, hallucinations, tremor, diaphoresis, agitation, seizure	IVF Benzodiazepines Barbiturates Propofol
Malignant Hyperthermia	**Volatile anesthetics, succinylcholine**	Minutes-hours	Autonomic instability, elevated CO2, **hyperthermia (may be late or not present)**, delirium	IVF Propofol **Dantrolene**
Neuroleptic malignant syndrome	Antipsychotics, dopamine withdrawal	Several days	Autonomic instability, delirium, **"lead pipe rigidity"**	IVF Benzodiazepines Propofol **Dopamine agonists such as Bromocriptine**
Serotonin syndrome	SSRI, SNRIs, **DXM, Tramadol, MAOIs, Lithium**	Hours	Autonomic instability, delirium, diarrhea, diaphoresis, mydriasis, hyperthermia, **hyperreflexia/clonus (LE prominent)**	IVF Benzodiazpines Barbiturates Propofol Cyproheptadine
Sympathomimetic	Cocaine, amphetamines, stimulants, cathinones	Hours	Tachycardia, hypertension, hyperthermia, delirium, seizure, mydriasis, **diaphoresis**	IVF Benzodiazepines Barbiturates Propofol

Toxic Threats

ARACHNIDS

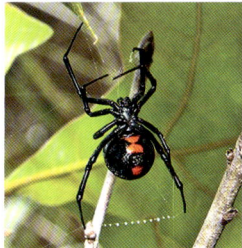
Black Widow

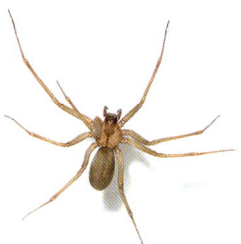
Brown Recluse

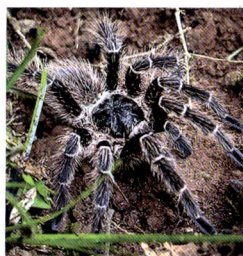
Tarantula

MARINE THREATS

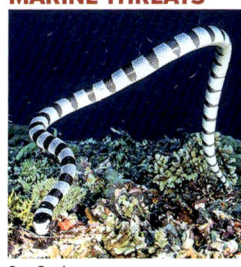
Sea Snake

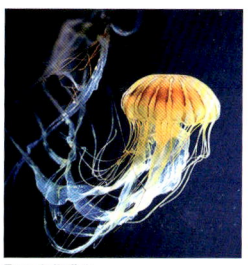
True Jellyfish

MARINE THREATS (CONT.)

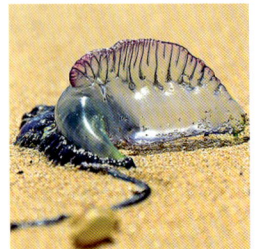
Portuguese Man o'War Jellyfish

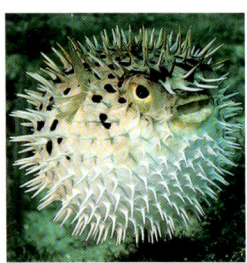
Pufferfish

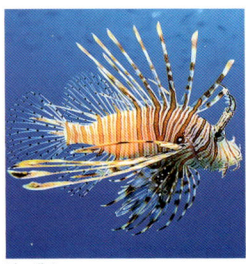
Lionfish

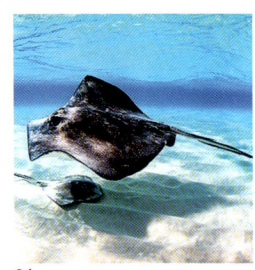
Stingray

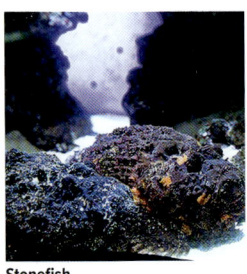
Stonefish

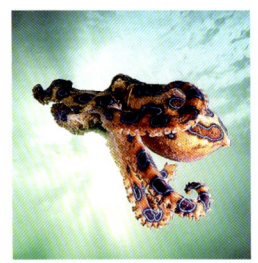
Blue-Ringed Octopus

MUSHROOMS

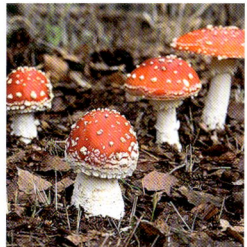

Amanita Muscaria

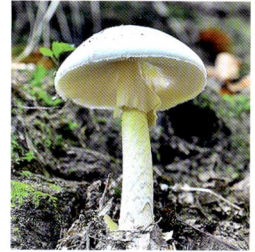

Amanita Phalloides

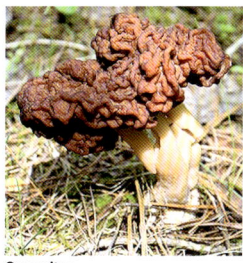

Gyromitra

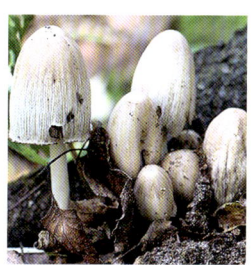

Inky Cap

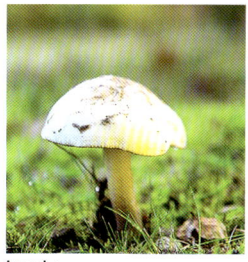

Inocybe

MUSHROOMS (CONT.)

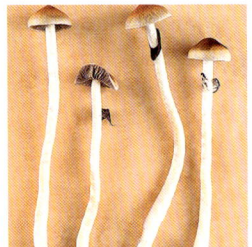
Psilocybe

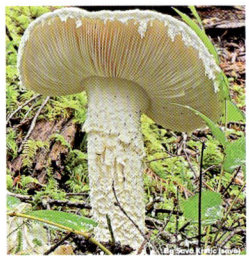
Amanita Smithiana

PLANTS

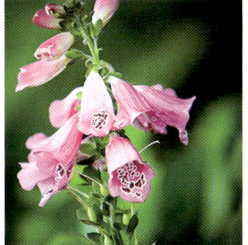
Digitalis

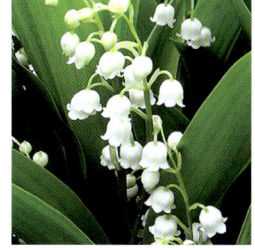
Lily of the Valley

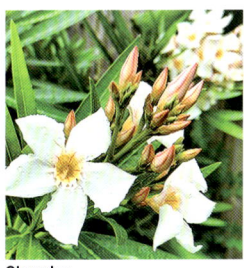
Oleander

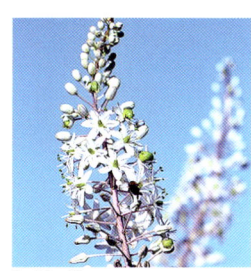
Red Squill

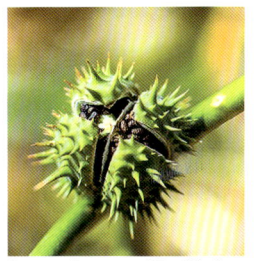
Datura—Jimsonweed Seed Pod

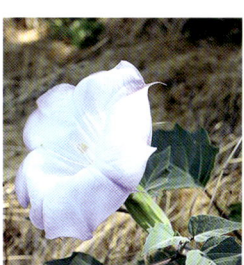
Datura—Jimsonweed

PLANTS (CONT.)

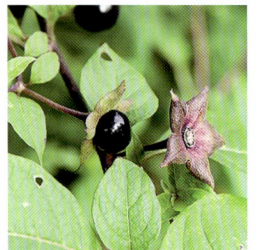

Deadly Nightshade Atropa

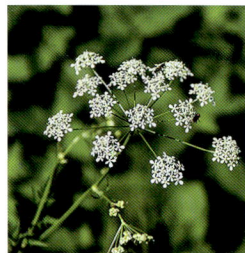

Water Hemlock

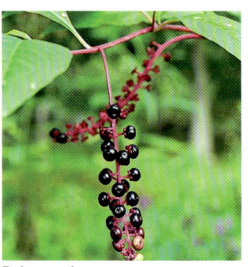

Pokeweed

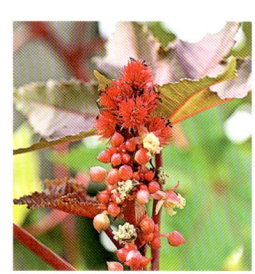

Ricin

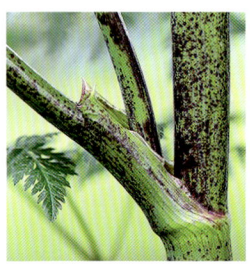

Poison Hemlock

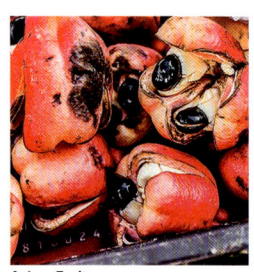

Ackee Fruit

PLANTS (CONT.)

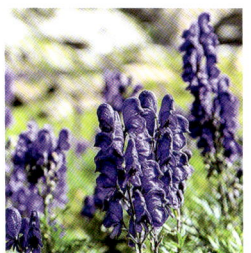
Aconite

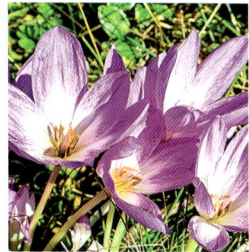
Colchicine

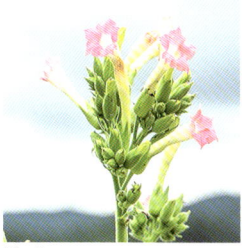
Nicotine

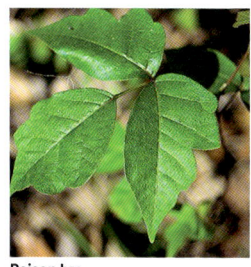
Poison Ivy

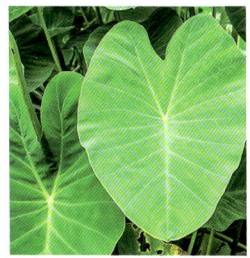
Elephant's Ear

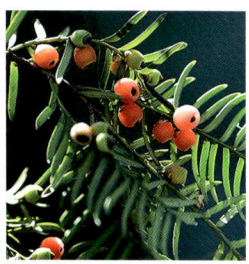
Yew

SNAKES

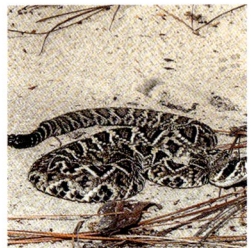
Eastern Diamondback

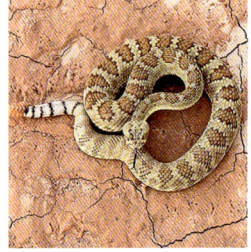
Mojave Rattlesnake

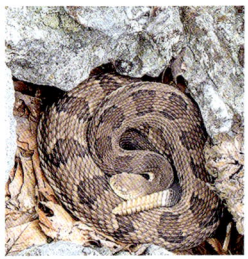
Timber Rattlesnake

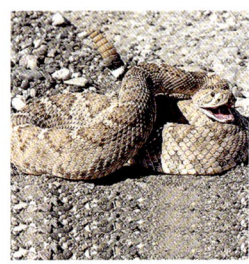
Western Diamondback

SNAKES (CONT.)

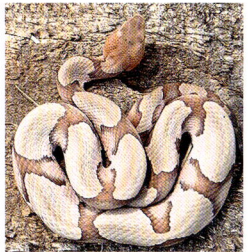
Copperhead

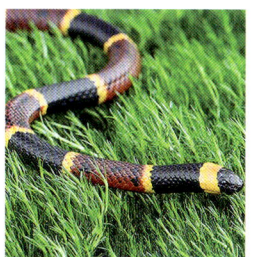
Coral Snake

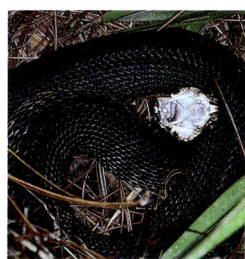
Cottonmouth (water moccasin)

STINGING INSECTS

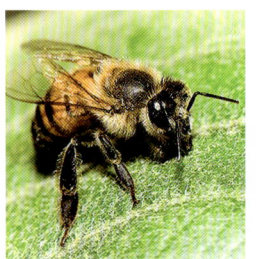
Africanized Honeybee

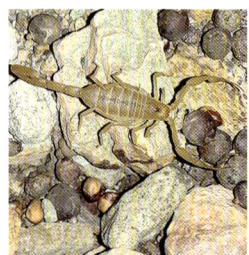
Bark Scorpion

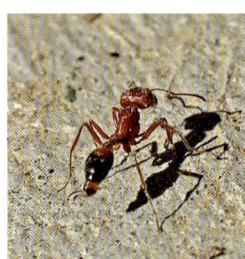
Fire Ant

LESIONS

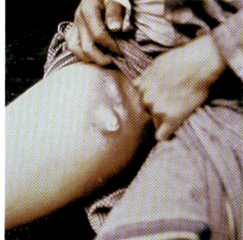
Bubonic Plague

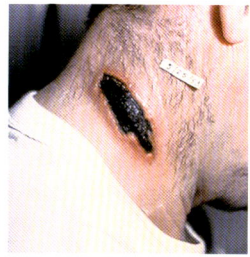
Cutaneous Anthrax

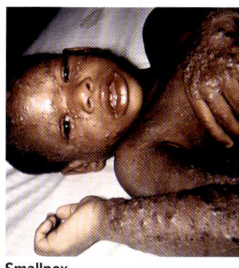
Smallpox

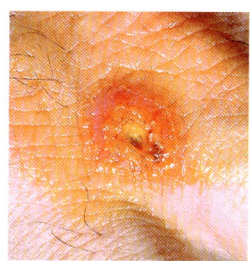
Tularemia

Images courtesy of CDC Public Health Image Library

Citations
References can be found at **emra.org/guides**.

Content Teams
Approach to the Poisoned Patient: Katz KD
Acetaminophen: Farber E, Romano TM, Kao LW
Alcohols-Ethanol: Allen J, Rosenau AM, Greller HA
Alcohols-Toxic: Bartlett KB, Goyke TE, Spyres MB
Anesthetics: Abbasi OZ, Burmeister DB, Schwarz ES
*Antibacterials: Dillon ZM, Cook M
Anticholinergics/Antihistamines: Daubert JW, Weaver KR, Kang AM
Anticoags-Heparin/Warfarin: Davis J, Quintana EC, Schwarz ES
Anticoags-DOACs/NOACs: Miller AJ, Barr GC Jr, Schwarz ES
Anticonvulsants: Dzike K, Youngdahl A, Kang AM
Antidepressants-TCAs/SSRIs/SNRIs/MAOIs: Amaducci AM, Goyke TE, Kopec K
Antidepressants-Lithium: Warren HR, Miller AC, Greller HA
Antidiabetics: Anderson RA, Cook M, Kang AM
Antidysrhythmics: Burket GA III, Cannon RD, Greller HA, Kopec K
Antihypertensives-Beta Blockers/CCBs: Bhimani SR, Kane BG, Spyres MB
Antihypertensives-ACEi/Alpha Agonists/Vasodilators: Ward HH, Kane BG, Schwarz ES
Antipsychotics-Atypical: Kailash P, Surmaitis RM, Schwarz ES
Antipsychotics-Typical: Gyory RA, Surmaitis RM, Greller HA
Caustics: Ely BJ, Amaducci AM, Gesell JM, Kao LW
Cholinergics: Day RS, Weaver KR, Kopec K
Digoxin: Fieman RE, Greenberg MR, Greller HA

Envenomations
Scorpions: Khan RA, Richardson DM
Vipers, Elapids: Makar GA, Sexton JD, Spyres MB
Arachnids, Hymenoptera: Fikse DJ, Coleman GA III, Spyres MB

Hallucinogens: Enyart J, Beauchamp GA, Greller HA
Hallucinogens-Ketamine/DXM: Frey AS, Beauchamp GA, Greller HA
Hemoglobinopathies: Goodheart V, Johnson SA, Kang AM
Heavy Metals: Wier AE, Yaeger SK, Kao LW
Hydrocarbons: Enyart J, Schwarz ES
Inhalants/Gas-Asphyxiants, HS, Aluminum Phosphide, Cyanide: Fritzges JA, Anderson RA, Carraro MN, Snow JW

Inhalants/Gas-Chlorine, NO: Gupta A, Roth KR, Snow JW
Marine Life: Marschall MD, Sexton JD, Spyres MB
Marijuana: Henry KA, Sclafani MJ, Kao LW
Methotrexate: Amaducci AM, Kang AM
Methylxanthines: Koons AL, MacKenzie RS, Greller HA
Mushrooms: Jong MR, Greller HA
Opioids: Kiernan EA, Kane KE, Schwarz ES
Opioids-Loperamide/Tramadol: Mason EK, Kane KE, Schwarz ES, Kopec K
Plants: Matuzsan ZM, Snow JW
Rodenticides: Yoder NM, Cannon RD, Snow JW
Salicylates: Amaducci AM, Kopec K
Sedative/Hypnotics: Maier JL, Martini WA Jr., Jacoby JL, Kopec K
Sympathomimetics: Melder RJ Jr., Johnson SA, Kopec K
Terrorism Agents: Collins DL, Nguyen MC, Kopec K
Terrorism-Radiation: Morolla LA, Nguyen MC, Kang AM
*Vitamins: Paulson CL, Greenberg MR
Common Formulas: Parikh PM, Chow R, Kang AM

Toxidromes
Anticholinergic: Sadowski J, Bean EW
Malignant Hyperthermia: Weaver KD, Eygnor JK
NMS: Parikh PM, Chow C
Serotonin Syndrome: Levi J, Quinn SM
Sympathomimetic: Palilonis MM, Dunn AL
Toxidromo Table: Katz KD

Withdrawal States
Ethanol: Urban CE, Worrilow CC, Spyres MB
Opiate/Opioid: Sheen AW, Evans EM, Kang AM
Sedative/Hypnotic: Tully BN, Worrilow CC, Spyres MB

*Chapter not included in print.

NOTES

NOTES

NOTES

NOTES

INDEX

2-PAM 279

A

ACE Inhibitors/ARB 154-156
Acetaminophe. 95-98
Acetaminophen Plasma
   Concentration 98
Acid, Hydrochloric 36-38
Acid, Hydrofluoric 38-42
Acid, Sulfuric 36-38
Acid, Valproic 127-128
Ackee Fruit 215-216, 288
Aconite (Aconitum) 218-219, 289
Africanized Honeybee 60-62, 292
Alcohols 9-18
Algorithm, Pit Viper Envenomation
   Management. 69-72
Alkali 35-36
Alpha-1 Antagonists 156-157
Alpha-2 Agonists 157-159
Alpha-Glucosidase Inhibitors 141
Aluminum Phosphide 201-203
Amphetamines 238-242
Amylin Analogs 142
Analogs, Amylin 142
Analogs, GLP-1 144-145
Andromeda 218-219
Anemone, Sea 50
Anesthetics, Local. 99-102
Anesthetics, Nitrous Oxide. 102
Angel's Trumpet (Brugmansia). ... 216
Anthrax 19-21, 293
Anti-hypertensives 154-167
Anticoagulants 108-116
Anticonvulsants 117-129
Antidepressant, Tricyclic 136-138

Antidepressants 129-140
Antidepressants, Atypical. 139-140
Antidiabetics 141-151
Antidotes. 270
Antidysrhythmics 103-108
Antidysrhythmics, Vaughan-Williams
   Classes 103-107
Antihistamines 151-154
Antimuscarinic Plants........... 216
Antimuscarinics 151-154
Antipsychotics. 167-172
Antipsychotics, Atypical 170-172
Antivenom, Black Widow 270
Antivenom, CroFab. 271
Antivenom, Sea Snake 280
Antivenom, Stonefish 280
APAP 95-98
Apixaban 108-109
Arachnids 57-60, 283
Aripiprazole. 170-172
Arsenic/Arsine. 73-75
Atropine 270
Atypical Antidepressants 139-140
Atypical Antipsychotics. 170-172
Autumn crocus 219-220, 289

B

Baclofen 197-198
Barbiturates 193-194
Barium. 206-207
Benzodiazepines 195-196
Beta Adrenergic
   Antagonists 159-162
Beta Blockers 159-162
Biguanides 142-143
Bioterrorism 19-34

Black Widow Antivenom 270
Black Widow Spider 57-58, 283
Blue-Ringed Octopus 43, 284
Botulism 21-23
Box Jellyfish 46-47
Bromocriptine.................. 271
Brown Recluse Spider 58-59, 283
Buprenorphine 181-190
Bupropion 139-140

C

Caffeine................... 178-181
Calcium...................... 271
Calcium Channel
  Antagonists..............162-164
Calcium Channel Blockers....162-164
Calcium EDTA 271
Cannabinoids, Synthetic 235-236
Carbamates 203-206
Carbamazepine 117-119
Carbon Monoxide............ 85-87
Cardiac Glycoside Plants 217
Cardiotoxic Sodium
  Blockers.................217-218
Cardiotoxic Sodium
  Channel Openers 218-219
Carfentanil 181-190
Carisoprodol...............196-197
Castor Bean 224
Cathinones 238-242
Caustics..................... 35-42
Chlorine...................251-252
Chlorpromazine 167-170
Chlorprothixene 167-170
Ciguatera 53-54
Clozapine 170-172

Cocaine...................238-242
Codeine................... 181-186
Colchicine 219-220, 289
Common Formulas.........269-270
Cone Snail...................... 44
CroFab Antivenom 271
Cyanide Antidote Kit............272

D

Dabigatran 109-111
Deadly Nightshade
  (Atropa bella-donna)......216, 288
Death Camas (Toxicoscordion
  venenosum) 218-219
Decontamination 4
Deferoxamine..................272
Dextromethorphan ..181-190, 227-228
Dextrose......................272
Diagnostics, General 5-6
Diazepam 272
Dieffenbachia 222
Digitalis......................286
Digoxin 172-176
Digoxin Specific FAB............272
Dimercaprol 270
Direct Oral Anticoagulants... 108-109
Disposition, General............ 7-8
Disposition, Hallucinogens/
  Psychotropics 233
Diuretics 165
DOACs................... 108-109
Dopamine 273
DPP-4 Inhibitors 144
Droperidol..................167-170
Drug Doses 270-281

302

E

ED Management of Alcohol
   Withdrawal Algorithm 263
Edoxaban 108-109
Elapidae 65-66, 290-291
Elephant's Ear 222, 289
Envenomations, Non-Marine . . . 57-72
Envenomations/Poisonings,
   Marine 43-56
Epinephrine 273
Esmolol 273
Ethanol (EtOH) 273
Ethanol 9-11
Ethanol Withdrawal 259-263
Ethylene Glycol 11-13

F

Fentanyl 181-186
Fire Ants 62-63, 292
Flame lily 219-220
Flumazenil 273
Fluoroacetamide 207-208
Fluphenazine 167-170
Folate 273
Fomepizole 274
Foxglove 217

G

Gabapentin 119
Gamma-Hydroxybutyrate 199
GHB 199
GI Decontamination 274
GLP-1 Analogs 144-145
Glucagon 274

H

Hallucinogens 227-233
Haloperidol 167-170
Haloperidol 275
Heavy Metals 73-83
Hemlock, Poison 220-221, 288
Hemlock, Water 221-222, 288
Hemoglobinopathies 85-89
Henbane (Hyoscyamus niger) 216
Heparin 111-113
Heroin 181-190
High-Dose Insulin
   Euglycemia 275
Hydrochloric Acid 36-38
Hydrocodone 181-190
Hydrofluoric Acid 38-42
Hydrogen Sulfide 252-254
Hydromorphone 181-190
Hydroxocobalamin 275
Hymenoptera 60-63, 292
Hypnotics 193-200
Hypoglycemics 141-151

I

Imidazopyridine 200
Indian Poke
   (Veratrum viride) 218-219
Indolealkylamines 232
Insoluble Oxalates 222
Insulin 145-147
Intravenous Lipid Emulsion 275
Iron 75-77
Irukandji Jellyfish 46-47
Isopropanol 13-14
Isoproterenol 275

J

Jamaican Vomiting
 Sickness 215-216
Jellyfish. 45-47, 283
Jequerity Bean 224
Jimsonweed (Datura
 stramonium) 216, 287

K

K2 235-236
Ketamine. 228, 275

L

L-carnitine. 276
Lacosamide. 120
Lamotrigine. 121-122
Lead 77-79
Leucovorin 276
Levetiracetam. 122-123
Lidocaine 276
Lily of the Valley 217, 287
Lionfish 48-50, 284
Lithium 129-131
Loperamide. 186-188
Lorazepam 276
LSD 229-230
Lysergamides (Natural). 228-229

M

Magnesium Sulfate. 276
Malignant Hyperthermia
 Syndrome 243-244
Mandrake 216
MAOIs 131-134
Marijuana 234-236
Marijuana, Synthetic. 234-236
Marine Envenomations/
 Poisonings. 43-56
Meglitinides 147-148
Meperidine 181-186
Mercury. 79-81
Mescaline .230
Metal Fume Fever. 81-82
Methadone 181-186
Methanol. 14-17
Methemoglobinemia 87-89
Methotrexate 176-178
Methylene Blue. 276
Methylxanthines 178-181
Monoamine Oxidase
 Inhibitors. 131-134
Morphine. 181-186
Mushrooms 91-94, 285-286

N

N-acetylcysteine. 277
Naloxone. .277
NDRIs .134-135
Neuroleptic Malignant
 Syndrome 245-247
New/Novel Oral
 Anticoagulants 108-109
Nicotine. 222-223, 237-238, 289
Nightshade (Atropa
 bella-donna) 216, 288
Nitrogen Dioxide. 255-256
NOACs. 108-109
Non-Marine Envenomations. . . . 57-72
Norepinephrine. 277
Norepinephrine Dopamine
 Reuptake Inhibitors. 134-135
Nutmeg 231

O

Octopus, Blue-Ringed 43
Octreotide 277
Olanzapine 170-172
Oleander 217, 287
Opiates 181-190
Opioid/Opiate Withdrawal . . . 264-265
Opioids 181-190
Opioids, Semi-Synthetic 181-190
Opioids, Synthetic 181-190
Organophosphates 203-206
Oxcarbazepine 117-119
Oxycodone 181-190
Oxymorphone 181-190

P

Paracetamol 95-98
Penicillamine 277
Pesticides 201-206
Phenobarbital 278
Phentolamine 278
Phenylephrine 278
Phenylethylamines 238-242
Phenytoin 123-124
Philodendron 222
Phosgene 256-257
Photo Index 283-291
Physostigmine 278
Phytonadione 281
Pimozide 167-170
Pit Viper Snakebite
    Management Algorithm 69-72
Pit Vipers 67-72, 290-291
Plague 23-25, 293
Plants 215-225
Plants, Antimuscarinic 216
Plants, Cardiac Glycosides 217
Poison Ivy 225, 289
Poison Oak 225
Poison Sumac 225
Pokeweed 223, 288
Portuguese Man o' War . . . 47-48, 284
Potassium Iodide 279
Pralidoxime Chloride 279
Pregabalin 124-125
Promethazine 167-170
Propofol 279
Propylene Glycol 17-18
Protamine Sulfate 279
Prothrombin complex
    concentrate 278
Prussian Blue 279
Psychotropics 227-233
Pufferfish 56, 284
Pyridoxine 279

Q

Quetiapine 170-172

R

Radiation 25-29
Rat Poison 206-213
Red Squill 217, 287
Rhododendron 218-219
Ricin 29-31, 288
Risperidone 170-172
Rivaroxaban 108-109
Rodenticides 206-213
Rosary Pea 224

S

Salicylates 190-193
Salvia 231-232
Scombroid 55
Scorpion Immune F(ab')2 Equine
   Injection 280
Scorpionfish 48-50
Scorpions 63-65, 292
Sea Anemone 50
Sea Snake Antivenom 280
Sea Snakes 51-52, 283
Sedative 193-200
Sedative/Hypnotics
   Withdrawal 265-268
Selective Norepinephrine
   Reuptake Inhibitors 134-135
Selective Serotonin Reuptake
   Inhibitors 134-135
Semi-Synthetic Opioids 181-190
Serotonin Syndrome 247-249
SGLT-2 Inhibitors 148-149
Smallpox 31-32, 293
Snail, Cone 44
Snakes 51-52, 65-72, 290-291
Snakes, Copperheads 67-72, 291
Snakes, Coral 65-66, 291
Snakes, Cottonmouths 67-72, 291
Snakes, Rattlesnakes 67-72, 290
Snakes, Sea 51-52, 283
Snakes, Water Moccasins . . 67-72, 291
SNRIs 134-135
Sodium Bicarbonate 280
Sodium Monofluoroacetate . . 207-208
Spice 235-236
Spider, Black Widow 57-58, 283
Spider, Brown Recluse 58-59, 283
Spider, Tarantula 60, 283
Spiders 57-60, 283

SSRIs 134-135
Stingray 52-53, 284
Stonefish 48-50, 284
Stonefish Antivenom 280
Strychnine 209-210
Substances of Abuse 227-242
Succimer 280
Sufentanil 181-190
Sulfonylureas 149-150
Sulfuric Acid 36-38
Superwarfarin Ingestion
   Management Algorithm 213
Superwarfarins 210-213
Sympathomimetics 238-242
Syndromes, Malignant
   Hyperthermia 243-244
Syndromes, Serotonin 243-244
Syndroms, Neuroleptic
   Malignant 243-244
Synthetic Cannabinoids 235-236
Synthetic Opiates 181-190

T

Tarantula 60, 283
TCAs 136-138
Tetrodotoxin 56
Thallium 82-83
THC 234-235
Thebaine 181-186
Theobromine 178-181
Theophylline 178-181
Thiamine 281
Thiazolidinediones 150-151
Thionidazine 167-170
Tiagabine 125-126
Topiramate 126
Toxalbumins 224
Toxic Gas 251-257

Toxic Inhalants 251-257
Toxicodendron 225
Toxidrome Table 282
Tramadol. 188-190
Treatment, General. 7
Tricyclic Antidepressants 136-138
Trifluoperazine 167-170
Tryptamines 232
Tularemia 33-34, 293
Type I Antidysrhythmics 103-107
Type III Antidysrhythmics 107-108
Typical antipsychotics 167-170

U

U-4770. 181

V

Valproic Acid. 127-128
Vasodilators 165-167
Vigabatrin 128
Viperidae. 67-72, 290-291
Vipers 67-72, 290-291
Vitamin K1. 281

W

W-18. 181
Warfarin. 113-116
Withdrawal States. 259-268

Y

Yew Plant 217-218, 289

Z

Z Drugs 200
Zaleplon .200
Ziprasidone. 170-172
Zolpidem. 200
Zonisamide 129
Zopiclone 200